A Beginner's Guide to Evidence Based Practice in Health and Social Care Professions

A Beginner's Guide to Evidence Based Practice in Health and Social Care Professions

Helen Aveyard and Pam Sharp

Open University Press

Open University Press
McGraw-Hill Education
McGraw-Hill House
Shoppenhangers Road
Maidenhead
Berkshire
England
SL6 2QL

email: enquiries@openup.co.uk
world wide web: www.openup.co.uk

and Two Penn Plaza, New York, NY 10121-2289, USA

First published 2009
Reprinted 2011

A catalogue record of this book is available from the British Library

ISBN-13: 978-0-33-523603-9 (pb) 978-0-33-523602-2 (hb)
ISBN-10: 0-33-523603-0 (pb) 0-33-523602-2 (hb)

Library of Congress Cataloging-in-Publication Data
CIP data applied for

Typeset by RefineCatch Limited, Bungay, Suffolk
Printed in the UK by Bell and Bain Ltd, Glasgow

Mixed Sources
Product group from well-managed
forests and other controlled sources
www.fsc.org Cert no. TT-COC-002769
© 1996 Forest Stewardship Council

FSC

The *McGraw·Hill* Companies

Contents

Acknowledgements

The authors would like to thank the following individuals for their help during the writing of this book.

Jill Gregory

Angela Harper

Phil Harper

Introduction

This book is for you if you are:

- A student starting out or undertaking a pre-registration course in any of the health and social care professions
- A registered practitioner, who may be returning to post-qualification study or to clinical practice after a career break
- Anyone who feels clinically or professionally 'out of date' or has ever said *'I am not an academic . . . I am practical'* or *'I've always done it this way'*
- A practice assessor/mentor[1] who is supporting students in practice and aware of the need to use evidence in your daily practice and to role model best practice to your students.

You already know that:

- You are legally and professionally accountable for your practice once you are a registered practitioner.
- As a student you may be called to account to your university or institution of higher education.
- There is a large amount and type of information available.
- You need skills in order to find, understand and use information.
- In order to function safely and/or to be successful as a student (pre- or post-qualifying) or member of staff you need to know how to apply relevant information to your practice and in your written work.

So . . . where do you start?
You might feel that you do not know where to begin to use this evidence in your practice and learning or that when you try to it is too complicated or

---

[1] The term practice assessor/mentor will be used throughout to describe those who support learners in practice, a variety of terms are used throughout the professions such as: clinical educator, supervisor, practice educator/teacher, clinical tutor or instructor.

difficult. **This book** will lead you through this process at an introductory level in a jargon-free way.

Aim

The aim of this book is to explain evidence based practice and to present it as a topic that practitioners of all levels, including students, can relate to from the very start of their clinical experience and in their writing. Evidence based practice is of course a practical topic; however, we are aware that it is assessed in academic writing and is a substantial component in almost all marking criteria for those studying for a professional qualification in health and social care.

A Beginner's Guide To Evidence Based Practice provides a step-by-step approach to using evidence in practice in a practical and straightforward way.

Examples

We have tried to include examples that may be generally understood and by a range of professions as we all work within a wider team. We would ask that you read through the examples even if they don't relate directly to your profession and think about the message the example is giving.

How to get the most from this book

- Try and read the introductory chapters first as the book is presented in the order we think it should be read, but you can use the index if you have a particular issue you want to find out about.
- Assess your own learning style preference e.g. VARK assessment tool (Fleming and Mills 1992) available at http://www.vark-learn.com/english/index.asp.
- Use the glossary for explanations of words you are unfamiliar with.
- Work with a colleague or a student who is more confident in using evidence in practice.
- Get access to the internet and start practising 'searching' using relevant databases (don't leave it until you really need to find information quickly).
- Do some additional reading around the topic of evidence based practice.

- Contact your local health and social care librarian (through your work organisation or local university) for additional, practical training sessions. Some university libraries have specialist health and social care librarians.
- Don't give up if you find something difficult or don't understand it. Feel good about every new thing that you have learnt.

Use the symbols

Key information

Activity for you to do

Think point

1

What is evidence based practice?

Having clear reasons for your practice decisions and your care • Delivering the best possible care using the best available evidence • How do we know what is best practice? • Defining evidence based practice • Accountability • Clinical governance • Legal and ethical considerations • Litigation/ negligence • Components of evidence based practice • Evidence based practice and patient/client preference • In summary • Key points

 Simply put, evidence based practice is practice that is supported by a clear, up-to-date rationale, taking into account the patient/client's preferences and using your own judgement. If we practice evidence based practice then we are set to give the best possible care.

Sounds complicated? Then read on . . .

Having clear reasons for your practice decisions and your care

If you are *a **student*** starting out on a course in any of the health and social care professions, you are likely to be well aware of the need to be able to explain the care that you give both in practice and in the assignments you write. This is because patients and clients expect you, even as a student, to understand why you are caring for them in a particular way and to explain the reasons (or rationale) for the care you give. This becomes increasingly important as you gain experience and become the one who is planning care and making decisions relating to care, rather than carrying out the instructions of others.

In short, use of a good evidence base for our practice decisions and planning care is what distinguishes us as registered health and social care professionals from those in assistant roles.

As a *registered professional* you may be aware that your practice may not be as current as it could be and this can make you feel vulnerable or under-confident. You may not have been able to access professional development opportunities or you may be about to re-start study and want to find out how to use evidence in your academic work.

If you are a *practice assessor/mentor* supervising learners or a *practitioner* who is returning to work or study after a career break, you are likely to be even more aware of this need. You may feel lacking in skills to act as a role model for best practice and lack confidence in giving the reasons you can give for your practice to others.

Example: Imagine you are a student studying social work and are out with your practice assessor/mentor. You visit a child who is known to be at risk of abuse and your practice assessor/mentor has to assess the immediate risk and decide whether to remove the child from the home. You ask your practice assessor/mentor how (s)he makes this decision. Your practice assessor/mentor explains to you how this assessment is made and gives you a clear rationale for the way (s)he has acted.

Example: Now imagine yourself or a family member arriving at the accident and emergency department with a swollen arm which you cannot move very well. The student practitioner on duty asks you to elevate your arm whilst you wait to see the duty doctor. It is painful for you to do this and you ask why it is necessary. Unfortunately, the student cannot tell you why you should elevate your arm. (S)he just says it's what they tell all patient/clients to do and that they have always told patient/clients to do this. The student is not aware of any evidence or rationale for the care and advice they give. How confident would you be in the care given in this department?

You can see from these simple examples that as a student or registered member of staff, it is essential that you can provide a clear rationale for the care you give. You need to be able to tell the patient/client/student why an intervention or procedure is required and be able to provide a clear rationale. This is part of evidence based practice.

But this alone is not enough

Being able to provide a clear rationale for the care you give is essential but not quite sufficient.

 Your rationale must be **clear** but it must also be **up to date and based on the best available evidence**.

This will enable you to develop the best possible evidence based practice. In the examples given earlier, the social worker needs to be aware of the evidence concerning when it is best practice to remove a child from their home. The student nurse needs to be aware of the evidence about post-trauma care. Usually, but not always, the evidence you use will come from **research**. Research into the outcomes of children at risk of abuse and post-trauma care will help us to work out what is best practice. But the research will come in many different forms and it is important that you recognise which evidence you need to base your practice on. We will discuss these different forms of evidence throughout this book.

Delivering the best possible care using the best available evidence

The main reason why you need to base your professional practice on the best available evidence (evidence based practice) is that it enables us to deliver the best possible patient/client care rather than out-of-date practice. Let's provide an example of what we mean.

Example: Let's say you go to a practitioner to enquire about the vaccinations required before you go abroad on a tropical holiday. Unfortunately, the practitioner is not up to date with current practice and recommends a vaccine which is now rarely used and has been largely replaced by a newer vaccine which has been found to be far more effective. The practitioner has been administering this older vaccine for years and is unaware of the newer more effective vaccination. They are therefore not practising evidence based practice because they are not using the best up-to-date evidence to inform their practice. Meanwhile your friend, who is travelling with you, visits a different practitioner and is given the new vaccine.

You experience some unpleasant side effects and when you read up about the vaccine, you discover that your friend is better protected than you are against the disease in question – and did not experience any side effects! You feel angry and your trust in the professional who had not given you the most up-to-date and best available health care is broken.

How do we know what is best practice?

This is where we need **evidence.** And it must be good evidence. You can see that tradition or acting because something is expected of you is not enough. In most cases, what we consider to be 'best practice' is determined by available **research evidence.** In the example given above, the newer vaccine will have been found to be more effective through research. In order to test effectiveness of a new vaccine (or any other drug or intervention) the best way to do this is usually by a **randomised controlled trial (RCT)** in which the new vaccine is given to one group of people, whilst the other established vaccine is given to another group of people and the effectiveness of both vaccines in preventing the disease in addition to any side effects experienced will be compared.

There are many different approaches to research and we will consider these as we continue working through this book. However, it is important to note that it is **research** that often – but not always – provides the **rationale** or **evidence** upon which we base our practice. There are many different types of research which we will consider throughout this book and we will discuss how different types of research are needed for different types of situation.

It will sometimes be the case that there is **not sufficient research evidence** upon which to base practice, or you find that the research evidence is inconclusive. It might also be unethical to undertake research to explore the area you are interested in. There will also be times when you need evidence other than research evidence. We will discuss this further as we go through this book.

Defining evidence based practice

We will now consider the concept of evidence based practice in more detail.

Evidence based practice is a term that has gained much popularity and attention in recent years. Simply put, evidence based practice is practice that is supported by clear reasoning, taking into account the patient's or client's preferences and using your own judgement.

It is a complex issue that has been defined and redefined as practitioners and academics debate their definitions. One of the most widely quoted and earliest definitions comes from David Sackett, founder of the NHS Research and Development Centre for Evidence Based Medicine in Oxford:

Evidence based practice is: 'the conscientious, explicit, and judicious use of current best evidence in making decisions about the care of individual patient/ clients' (Sackett *et al.* 1996 pp.71–72).

Here, Sackett helps us to understand that there is a strong link between evidence based practice and the decisions we make in our everyday practice and that our decisions should be clearly stated (explicit) and well-thought through (judicious), and use evidence sensibly and carefully.

In a more recent definition Dawes *et al.* (2005 p.7) in the Sicily statement offers a softer more holistic definition of evidence based practice:

Evidence Based Practice (EBP) requires that decisions about health and social care are based on the best available, current, valid and relevant evidence. These decisions should be made by those receiving care, informed by the tacit and explicit knowledge of those providing care, within the context of available resources.

This definition is interesting because it places the onus for the decision making with the patient/client rather than purely with the health or social care professional. It also recognises that we draw on hidden or intuitive (tacit) knowledge as well as that which we can explain.

Where do you think the balance should lie between the health and social care provider making a decision and that decision being made by those in receipt of care?

Thompson *et al.* (2005) provide the following **staged approach** to illustrate evidence based practice:

1 Identify a clinical question in response to a recognised information need.
2 Search for the most appropriate evidence.
3 Critically appraise this evidence.
4 Incorporate the evidence into a strategy for action.
5 Evaluate the effects of any decisions and action taken.

Although delivery of the **best possible care** is the main driver behind evidence based practice, there are other reasons why it is important to be able to explain your care decisions and these will now be discussed.

Accountability

As a health or social care professional, you are **accountable**. This means that you must be able to justify, give a clear account of and rationale for your practice. Failure to do this can result in professional misconduct.

In the example given earlier, you might feel like making a complaint against the practitioner who gave you the out-of-date vaccine, especially if it caused you to have unpleasant side effects or reduced your enjoyment of the holiday by fearing that you were not fully protected by the vaccination. If you did make a complaint, the practitioner would then have to justify why this out-of-date vaccine was given.

- Students are accountable to their higher education institution and when in practice should be supervised by a registered professional.
- Registered practitioners are accountable to their professional body and their employers.
- We are all accountable to the law.

If there was a standard or policy document in his or her place of work that recommended the newer vaccine, then the practitioner would find it difficult to justify administering the old vaccine. Even if no such documentation existed, the practitioner would still find it difficult to justify why an outdated vaccine was administered when a more effective vaccine with fewer side effects was available.

We can see that when you are called to account for your practice, you will only be able to do so if you have administered care that is based on the best available evidence. You will not be able to account for care that is based on old or weak evidence.

Find out what your **professional body, college** or **association** says about your accountability and evidence based practice.

In the United Kingdom these are as follows:

For occupational therapists, physiotherapists, operating department practitioners, dieticians, paramedics, radiographers, speech and language therapists, art therapists, chiropodists/podiatrists, clinical scientists, orthoptists, prosthetists and orthotists: the **Health Professions Council (HPC)**. They publish their Standards of Conduct, Performance and Ethics (2008) available at http://www.hpc-uk.org/aboutregistration/standards/.

They state that 'you must keep your professional knowledge and skills up to date' (HPC 2008 p.10).

For nurses: the **Nursing and Midwifery Council (NMC)**. They publish their Standards of Conduct, Performance and Ethics (2008) available at http://www.nmc-uk.org/aSection.aspx?SectionID=45.

This most recent NMC Code for Nurses and Midwives came into effect on 1 May 2008 and requires all practitioners to deliver evidence based care. Practitioners are required to 'provide a high standard of care and practice at all times' and to 'deliver care based on the best available evidence or best practice' (NMC 2008 p.7).

The Code declares nurses and midwives to be accountable for the care they deliver: 'you are personally accountable for actions and omissions in your practice and must always be able to justify your decisions' (NMC 2008 p.1).

Therefore, if you are called upon to account for your practice, you must be able to provide a sound rationale for why you acted as you did. If you are only able to say '*I was told to do this*' or '*I've always done it this way*', your practice will look very poor indeed! Students are expected to work towards these standards in order to obtain registration and failure to do so may affect progression towards qualification.

Do you think the practitioner referred to earlier would be found guilty of professional misconduct because of the decision to administer a vaccine which had been superseded by a more effective vaccine? Would that verdict have been reached if he/she had used an evidence based approach to the selection of the appropriate vaccine?

Individual colleges or associations may also be involved in setting professional guidance (see Appendix: Useful websites).

Clinical governance

In the United Kingdom, clinical governance is defined through the *National Health Service*, the Department of Health website, which states that:

'Clinical governance is the system through which NHS organisations are accountable for continuously improving the quality of their services and safeguarding high standards of care, by creating an environment in which clinical excellence will flourish.'

Available at http://www.dh.gov.uk/en/Publichealth/Patientsafety/Clinical governance/DH_114.

Clinical governance is often described as an umbrella term incorporating several aspects relating to maintaining quality, professional development and risk management. There is a **National Clinical Audit** which is a quality improvement process. Clinical audit and outcomes measurements are quality improvement tools that can help to close the gap between what is known to be the best care and the care that patient/clients are receiving. They aim to ensure that all patient/clients receive the most effective, up-to-date and appropriate treatments, delivered by clinicians with the right skills and experience. Clinical audit against good practice criteria or standards answers the question – are patient/clients given the best care? Clinical outcomes measurement answers the questions – are they better, and do they feel better?

The **Essence of Care** benchmarking statements 'The essence of care' have been designed to support the measures to improve quality set out by the DH (1998) in *A First Class Service*, and aim to contribute to the introduction of clinical governance at local level. The benchmarking process outlined in 'The essence of care' helps practitioners to take a structured approach to sharing and comparing practice, enabling them to identify the best practice and to develop action plans to remedy poor practice.

These documents are available at http://www.dh.gov.uk/en/Publichealth and social/Patient/clientsafety/Clinicalgovernance/index.htm.

Standards and quality assurance initiatives will be present in non-NHS organisations too.

Legal and ethical considerations

As registered practitioners you are personally responsible for your practice and accountable to the law, your professional body and your employer. This is under the following areas:

*   Criminal liability (in a Crown Court)
*   Civil liability (negligence and liability to pay compensation)
*   Professional liability (codes of conduct and ethics)
*   Employment (contract of employment).

(Dimond 2008)

Litigation/negligence

Another reason why it is important that you can justify the care that you give is that this may protect you or your organisation from litigation. There is a developing culture of litigation and claims against health and social care organisations. Patients or clients who are unhappy about the care they receive can make a claim in negligence if they have suffered harm as a result of that care. There is a National Health Service Litigation Authority (NHSLA) that deals with such claims and the NHS Redress Bill 2005 states that patient/clients who suffer as a result of NHS mistakes could receive up to £20,000 compensation without going to court. Clinical governance, discussed later, includes several measures to ensure we provide safe and effective care.

Let's return to the example about the administration of an outdated travel vaccination. Let's say that the worst does happen and you contract a serious tropical disease whilst you are away, the disease against which you had been vaccinated (with the less effective vaccine). Your travelling companion does not contract the disease. You become very ill and lose sight in one eye and are unable to work. In order to seek compensation you make a claim of negligence against the health care provider who did not use the best available evidence when selecting your travel vaccinations.

To make a successful claim in negligence against a health and social care provider, the patient/client has to demonstrate that the health care provider failed in their duty to provide care and that this failure led to harm. The courts have consistently ruled that such a failure occurs if the health or social care provider has not provided care that is evidence based. Evidence suggests that, in this case, the administration of an outdated vaccine less effective than its newer version led to a greater likelihood of your contracting the disease and might lead to a claim of negligence. Under the current system, you can only make a claim in negligence if you have suffered harm. Therefore, you would not be able to claim in negligence just because you had received the less effective vaccine; you would only be able to make a claim if you did contract the disease.

Let's then say that unfortunately your friend also contracts the disease, despite receiving the newer vaccine – (no vaccination is ever 100% effective). If (s)he then attempts to bring a case in negligence against the health and social care provider, (s)he is less likely to be able to succeed because the practitioner in this case used the most up-to-date evidence to select the appropriate vaccine and hence did not fail in the duty owed to the patient/client.

You can see that being able to provide a good rationale or explanation for your practice is an essential component of the concept 'evidence based practice' and might even prevent you from becoming involved in any legal proceedings.

Therefore, you can see that you are less likely to make errors or give the wrong information to your service users if you follow recommendations for best practice and have a sound rationale for what you do. We will now return to exploring in more detail what evidence based practice entails.

Components of evidence based practice

There are three main components of evidence based practice:

- Use of evidence.
- Clinical or professional judgement.
- Patient/client preference.

The availability of resources may also need to be considered at the implementation stage.

We have discussed the use of evidence and will be returning to this throughout this book. We will now explore the use of clinical or professional judgement and patient/client preference.

Evidence based practice and clinical/professional judgement

As we have already mentioned, evidence alone is not enough for evidence based practice. Our own clinical judgement is also vital for assisting with providing an evidence based approach to care. This is because the evidence that we find does not refer to the specific patient/client we are looking after and a judgement is needed as to the relevance of the evidence we have to the particular **context** and the **individual** patient or client.

Sometimes you might hear people say *'evidence based practice is too rigid and doesn't relate to my own clinical experience and professional judgement'*.

This should not be the case!

All those who believe in and promote evidence based practice agree that research evidence alone is not enough to inform our practice. Individual expertise of the practitioner is required to apply the evidence in an appropriate way, using their clinical or professional judgement.

At other times you might hear people say *'Well I use my intuition and experience, I have been practising for 25 years. I don't need evidence based practice.'*

This also should not be the case!

People often talk about the intuition involved when experienced practitioners deliver care. Evidence based practice is not an alternative to the use of intuition. Instead intuition is incorporated into evidence based practice when clinical or professional judgement is applied.

According to Benner and Tanner (1987) intuitive knowledge and analytical reasoning are not opposed to each other – they can and do work together.

* Intuition is often referred to as gut feeling (just knowing).
* There appears to be a close relationship between experience and intuition.
* Intuition is grounded in both knowledge and experience in making judgements.

(Benner 1984; Benner and Tanner 1987)

This is not an excuse to use our experience or intuition alone, but that judgement should be used alongside the evidence or used when there is no available evidence, conflicting evidence or poor quality evidence. We should of course recognise areas where we lack experience or expertise.

Sackett, one of the founders of evidence based practice, describes how evidence can inform decisions about practice, but cannot replace clinical expertise and judgement. He argues that clinical expertise is used to determine whether the available evidence should be applied to the individual patient/client at all and, if so, if it should be used to inform our clinical decision making (Sackett *et al.* 1996).

So what do we mean by clinical/professional judgement?

In order to make sound decisions for our professional practice we need to know what options are available to inform our care/practice decisions. In the first instance we need evidence upon which to base our decision. This is normally, but not always, research based evidence. However we also need to use our clinical judgement to make the right decision. Clinical judgement uses our own previous experiences and knowledge of the patient/client and local surroundings, in order to make a decision about clinical care. Many health and social care practitioners state that their **professional work is an art as well as a science** and it incorporates a human element which cannot be reduced to just the application of research knowledge to patient/client care. This can be described as clinical or professional judgement.

 In summary, evidence based practice requires more than 'raw' evidence. It requires clinical or professional judgement, intuition and experience so that the evidence is appropriately applied in practice.

Evidence based practice and patient/client preference

So far we have established that available evidence needs to be combined with clinical or professional judgement in applying evidence based practice. There is also a third component – that the patient/client's preference must be acknowledged and their **consent** sought prior to the undertaking of any intervention.

If all the best evidence and clinical or professional judgement pointed towards an intervention that the patient/client did not accept, then we could not carry it out.

This is because all care delivered must be with the agreement or consent of the patient/client. Any care that is delivered without the patient/client's consent may be unlawful. The exceptions to this are if it is an emergency or the patient/client is unable to consent. In these cases, care for patient/clients should be delivered that is in their best interests. This requirement for consent is a legal requirement which reinforces the importance of information giving prior to all care procedures as an individual cannot make decisions about the choices offered to them without full information about the options available to them. The **Discern** website (2008) offers guidelines for producing and reviewing patient/client information available at http://www.discern.org.uk/discern_instrument.php.

Find out what your own professional body says about obtaining consent.

Successive governments have put patient/client choice and involvement in decision making (DH 2004) high on their agenda and some patient/clients really want to be involved in the decisions relating to their care. Others will trust that the professional will make the best possible decision on their behalf. This is a big responsibility and we need to be well informed as to what is the best for our patient/clients. The Department of Health (2004a) note that patient/client involvement is often tokenistic and in reality health and social care professionals 'decide' what decisions patient/clients can be involved in. They recommend that health and social care professionals should anticipate 'decision making situations' and develop awareness of joint decision making processes.

You can assist your patient/client in their decision making by helping them to clarify:

• The decision they need to make

- Their decision making needs
- Their support needs
- Their knowledge needs/certainty
- Their values and relationship with benefits/risk.

There is a useful decision making guide available at http://decisionaid.ohri.ca/decguide.html.

Whilst formal consent is often not sought prior to care procedures and the law recognises the role of implied consent, an implied consent prior to care can only be considered to be valid if prior information has been given to the patient/client (Aveyard 2004). It is therefore vital for professionals to become confident and competent in information giving.

If the patient/client is not able to consent to care (for example in an emergency or if the patient/client has a condition which inhibits his or her ability to consent) then you have a professional duty to deliver the care that is in the patient/client's best interests. In this instance, the patient/client's best interests would be determined using the best available evidence and clinical or professional judgement only.

The Mental Capacity Act 2005 (implemented 2007)

- Presumes capacity
- Reinforces the right of individuals to be supported to make decisions
- Reinforces the right of individuals to make eccentric or unwise decisions
- Reinforces that anything done for or on behalf of people without capacity must be done 'in their best interests'
- Reinforces that anything done for or on behalf of people without capacity should be least restrictive of rights and freedoms.

Available at http://www.publications.parliament.uk/pa/cm200304/cmbills/120/04120.1–4.html#j02.

It is important to remember that the final component of evidence based practice is that of determining patient/client preference. Care cannot be delivered without the consent of the patient/client and if you do not gain consent as a practitioner, you are at risk of professional misconduct and in breach of the law.

What does evidence based practice mean to me?

Example: You have a question about something you do in everyday practice, or you may have noticed that several practitioners carry out an intervention or go about a case study differently.

Example: You have been asked to write an essay or discuss a case study on a given scenario discussing what you did and why you did it.

For both examples you would need to ask the question: '*What is the evidence for this intervention?*'

First of all, you need to **search for** and **locate** the appropriate evidence. You might find a wide range of different research studies, case studies, guidelines, literature reviews or opinion articles. You would then need to **judge the quality** of the evidence you find and if it is relevant to your problem or issue. You would probably consider any research that you find to be of more value than someone's personal view. This evidence should then be **applied** to the care of the patient/client whose needs initiated the clinical question, taking into account their preference and your clinical or professional judgement. The **resources** available may also need to be considered at this point. You may then want to **evaluate** the effectiveness of your intervention in that situation with that patient/client.

We will consider asking the right question, searching for the evidence, and judging the value and quality of different types of evidence in more detail later in this book.

This is evidence based practice in practice!

In summary

In this chapter we have discussed the meaning of the term evidence based practice. We hope that you are now thinking that there is a good logical argument for health and social care to be evidence based. After all, who would want to receive outdated care from a professional who could not account for it in preference to care that is based on the best available evidence combined with professional judgement?

In the remainder of this book we will consider why practice needs evidence and what we mean by evidence. We will then consider different research approaches that you might encounter. We will discuss how to search for evidence and then to consider how to determine whether it is any good or not. Before that we will consider in more detail why evidence based practice has become so important in our practice today.

Key points

1 There are several reasons why we need to adopt evidence based practice
   i   to ensure best practice
   ii for our professional accountability
   iii to avoid litigation/negligence claims.

2 Evidence based practice incorporates using best available evidence, clinical or professional judgement and patient/client preference in our decision making.
3 Evidence based practice does not replace using intuition or experience in our practice.

2

The development of evidence based practice

The information revolution • Why is there so much information available?
• So how does this 'information revolution' affect me? • Where do I find
this information? • Will I always find up-to-date research and information
for my practice? • How can I increase the chance of finding relevant
information for my practice? • In summary • Key points

In this chapter we will:

- Explore the arrival of evidence based practice
- Discuss how this has superseded the role of tradition and ritual in our practice within health and social care.

So far we have argued that evidence based practice is an important and essential approach to the delivery of health and social care. We have discussed how evidence based practice is practice which is based upon a sound, up-to-date rationale, your own clinical or professional judgement and taking into account the patient/client's wishes. We have also discussed how as a student or registered professional you need to be able to give reasons for the care you deliver. These are some of the reasons why evidence based practice has become so important in recent years.

It probably seems sensible and logical to you as you read this book that practice should be based on evidence where possible. However, it is important to acknowledge that evidence based practice is a relatively new concept. This is because research is a relatively new concept and prior to the advent of research knowledge, practitioners had little evidence upon which to base their care.

 For many centuries, the concept of **tradition and ritual** dominated health and social care.

You might imagine that life was much easier for our counterparts in days gone by who did not have to seek a research based rationale prior to delivering care nor did they have to access and interpret all the available knowledge on a particular topic.

 Think about how much easier it must have been in the days before there was much available evidence upon which to base health and social care. Maybe there was one key handbook for you to read, rather than the many journals that are now relevant to your professional field.

Practitioners in days gone by largely relied on trial and error, experience, ritual and what was accepted practice to inform the delivery of care. You are probably familiar with some popular rituals that were often practised.

 Think back to practices that you have previously carried out that are now considered unhelpful or even harmful. If you are a student ask your practice assessor/mentor.

Let's take some examples of practices which have been carried out and which do not have an evidence base to support them.

In many countries, children born to unmarried mothers were removed from their mothers and placed in temporary care. Here convention and social norms of the time were considered more important than the needs of the child and mother. The importance of the mother–child relationship was not considered significant.

In some countries, there used to be the practice of administering blood to newborn babies via the umbilical cord. It was thought that the administration of blood to the newborn would enhance and stimulate growth. In fact there was no evidence that this would be the case and as a result thousands and thousands of babies became infected with blood borne infections such as human immunodeficiency virus (HIV).

From these examples, you can see that absence of an appropriate evidence base led to practices that we would now consider very harmful.

Let's consider a less serious example – that of adding salt to the bathwater of patient/clients with wounds, or rubbing the area surrounding a pressure sore to increase the blood flow and hence the rate of healing. When research was undertaken to explore the effectiveness of these practices, it was found that adding salt to the bath had no influence on the rate of wound healing and rubbing the delicate area of skin around a pressure sore to be harmful to the patient/client. These practices are therefore no longer undertaken.

In the area of child protection, there has been recent criticism of practices and policies which have left children living in known high risk situations. Much research is now being undertaken to explore the presumption that children should be left in their home situation as long as possible and when or whether it is advisable to remove them from their homes. We need high quality evidence to make these decisions. Relying on tradition or accepted practice is no longer acceptable.

Can you identify an area of your own profession, where practice has changed due to new treatments or interventions?

Some examples of evidence that has led to changes in practice

The introduction of evidence based practice has led to a move away from practices that are based on tradition and for which there is no evidence based rationale.

Example: Take the following example which comes from the medical treatment of breast cancer but is used here as it illustrates the points we are making. If we look back 50 years, the best known treatment for breast cancer was a full mastectomy, which entailed the total removal of the breast. This was the standard treatment for many years. In the 1970s scientists began to consider whether such radical treatment was indeed the best option and commenced trials to compare whether removal of the malignant lump would be as effective as removal of the whole breast. Many very large studies (known as randomised controlled trials – which we will explore in more detail later in this book) were conducted across Europe and within the United States of America and the results of these studies confirmed that in fact it was both safe and effective to remove just the lump rather than the whole breast. As a result of these many studies, practitioners were able to inform patient/clients that a full mastectomy was no longer necessary and the best possible treatment, in most instances became the removal of the lump only.

We can therefore see that as a result of these trials, it was possible to establish best practice for the management of breast cancer. The results of these trials led to radical changes in the way that breast cancer was managed.

Example: The precautions taken to prevent cross-infection in many clinical and social environments provide another example. Whilst hand-washing was considered for a long time to be the most effective way of hand decontamination, researchers began to explore whether hand-rubbing with an antiseptic agent/ alcohol gel would be as effective in reducing cross-infection as the more traditional hand-washing methods (Girou *et al.* 2002). Some research studies identified that hand-rubbing was as effective and also more convenient than hand-washing and as a result, most hospitals were supplied with hand-rubbing facilities for staff, patient/clients and their visitors. However, one thing we must always be aware of is that **evidence is always evolving** and subsequent research has identified that hand-rubbing is not effective against all viruses and bacteria and more recently, the use of hand-washing has once again been promoted. This illustrates that we must always be alert and receptive to new evidence about practice.

The information revolution

There is a vast amount of information available to health and social care practitioners. This information is also expanding on a daily basis.

Every day, a vast number of journals relating to many different specialties and topics publish many papers from researchers and leading experts. As increasing amounts of research and other information become more readily available, it is, at least in theory, possible to say with more and more certainty what amounts to good practice and what does not. Sometimes, this evidence is inconclusive and sometimes contradictory and as we shall see, you can be faced with an over-whelming amount of information to process. This problem is partially solved by the existence and popularity of **literature reviews**, which summarise all the relevant literature on a particular topic. We shall explore this later in this book.

It is also important to note that patient/clients themselves are aware of new developments and treatments from the easy access to the internet and wide media cover. Kirschning *et al.* (2007) and Ziebland *et al.* (2004) discuss how patient/clients use the internet for additional sources of information and second opinion about their treatment.

There are some well-advertised and easily available sources where the public can seek information, either as information leaflets produced by professional organisations or the internet for example:

British Broadcasting Corporation (BBC) health and social information available at http://news.bbc.co.uk/1/hi/health and social/default.stm

NHS Direct available at http://www.nhsdirect.nhs.uk/

Clinical Knowledge Summaries information for patient/clients available at http://www.cks.library.nhs.uk/information_for_patient/clients

Patient UK available at http://www.patient.co.uk/ which provides a wide range of information including translated and audio information.

There is also a vast amount of unconfirmed and less reliable information around. Goldacre (2008) illustrates this in his book entitled *Bad Science*. In this book, Goldacre identifies the many myths that are around, most of which involve health and social care and demystifies them by citing the available evidence upon which the myths are based, for example, the whole area of detoxification, upon which much money and consumerism is based. Goldacre notes the lack of quality evidence that there is any such thing as detoxification and illustrates how evidence has not been used to back up the claims made by those advocating the 'science' of detoxification. It is clearly within your role as a health and social care professional to get behind the evidence so that you are not supporting claims that do not have a scientific basis.

Why is there so much information available?

There are two main reasons as to why there is so much available evidence:

- Increased demand for research and more/better quality research is produced.
- Information is more widely available from the internet.

Increased demand for research and more/better quality research is produced

Although evidence based practice is often described as a new idea within health and social care, it has gradually grown since the 1970s. At this time, practitioners increasingly began to search for a rationale for the care they delivered which previously might have been given according to tradition and experience. More professions have moved towards university education rather than on-the-job training or apprenticeship. With this, there has been an increase in the amount and quality of professional research. However, then came the realisation that whilst research and evidence for practice was available, this was not being incorporated into practice. The so-named **theory–practice divide** emerged. In order to overcome this, evidence based practice became a strategy for getting research into practice. So whilst the term evidence based practice is nothing particularly new, actually making it work in the reality of practice requires a range of approaches.

Over time, the term 'research based practice' gradually became replaced by the term 'evidence based practice' which emphasises the need for clinical or professional judgement and consideration of patient/client preferences to be used with the application of best available research findings or other evidence.

As the concept of evidence based practice has developed, you are also likely to come across many names that describe evidence based practice. The main thing to remember is that the idea behind evidence based practice is the same.

Some of the other terms that are used to refer to evidence based practice:

Evidence based medicine, Research based practice, Evidence informed practice

Evidence based nursing, Evidence based physiotherapy, Evidence based dietetics

Evidence based midwifery, Evidence based occupational therapy etc.

Information is more widely available from the internet

There has been a dramatic increase in **information technology** which has led to the increasing availability of information. Before the advent of this technology, libraries contained hard-bound indexes and volumes of the journals that were likely to be most relevant to their students. However, there were always a large number of journals unavailable to students or available only through inter-library loan. This meant that it was difficult and expensive to access relevant information. Nowadays, with the advent of online libraries, databases and journals, students and practitioners have access to many thousands of journals and books in addition to websites and other sources of information and references.

So how does this 'information revolution' affect me?

In short, as practitioners we have a duty to incorporate this information into our everyday practice to enhance patient/client care. As we have already discussed, practitioners are accountable for their practice and this requirement has grown with the increasing amount of information that is available regarding health and social care. As the available information increases, it is more and more likely that there will be some research available that underpins the care or treatment you deliver. Therefore if you deliver care as you have always done in the past without seeking to update yourself, it is likely that you will find that your practice is out of date and there is evidence to support a different practice or way of doing things. You may then be called to account for why your practice is out of date. Although practising health and social care today is more difficult than it was in previous times, it is even more important to keep up to date.

Where do I find this information?

In general, you will find the most up-to-date literature in the academic journals that are related to your subject or field. Your subject librarian at your university or hospital will be happy to guide you. You will find academic journals relating to a very wide range of professional interests. Some journals are generic to the interests of one professional group – for example *Journal of Clinical Nursing* or *British Journal of Occupational Therapy*, whilst others are specialist journals belonging to a particular area of professional interest for example *Addiction*. Academic journals contain many articles about different topics related to the overall subject addressed by the journal.

Journals often contain a mixture of research, literature reviews and discussion/ opinion articles, which we will discuss later on in this book in more depth.

You can **find journal articles** in a variety of ways:

- Accessing the journal archives via their website or sometimes a search engine on the internet
- Accessing an electronic library using the internet, with a password supplied by your librarian
- Accessing the paper copies (often referred to as hard copies) in your library.

Will I always find up-to-date research and information for my practice?

Whilst there has been a huge increase in the amount of available information, it is still the case that some areas of health and social care are under-researched. Research is still a developing area in some fields, and not all areas are under-pinned by a sound body of knowledge. So you might find yourself in one of two situations:

* You are bombarded by a wealth of information that you need to make sense of, or
* You do not find any information that relates to your selected topic.

We will discuss this further when we explore how to search for information and how to make sense of the information that you find later in this book.

How can I increase the chance of finding relevant information for my practice?

Throughout this book, we will explore how you can search for and evaluate information that you will need in your everyday practice. There are several things you can do to improve your chances of accessing the right information at the right time:

* Be clear and focussed on what you are looking for.
* Become familiar with approaches to searching and accessing information.
* Search for literature reviews initially rather than individual pieces of research.
* Be prepared to evaluate what you read.
* Set up email alerts so you get contents lists of the most relevant journals.
* Attend conferences.
* Invite specialist speakers to your workplace.
* Identify team members to specialise in one area.
* Set up a Journal club.
* Set up an evidence based practice group.

In summary

The advances in health and social care research which provide us with evidence for good practice, in combination with ever advancing communication technology has resulted in a huge amount of readily available information for health and social care professionals.

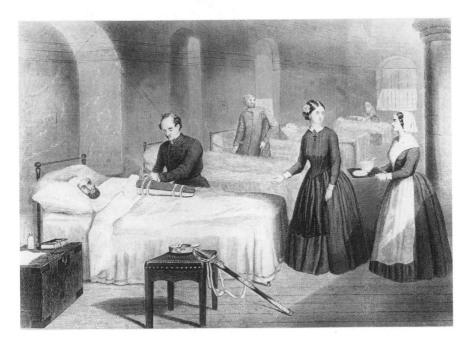

We can see how various factors have come together to bring about a revolution in the way in which we practise health and social care. No longer is it acceptable to say '*this is how I've always done this*' and to carry on with an outdated practice in the light of new evidence. The increase in the amount of available evidence and the ways that this can be accessed, together with the demand and drive for research evidence has led to an expectation and culture in which practice is founded on evidence and that you as a student or qualified practitioner need to be able to justify the care that you give.

In the remainder of this book, we will explore how you can best access, evaluate and make sense of the information that is available to you so that you can manage this in a way that facilitates you working within a culture of evidence based practice.

Key points

1 It is no longer acceptable to base our practice on tradition or ritual.
2 The dramatic rise in the quantity, quality and availability of information has led to the need to incorporate this information into daily practice.
3 Use of good quality, up-to-date evidence is expected by our patient/clients and we are accountable for ensuring we use it.

3

When do we need to use evidence and what evidence do we need?

Where to start – when do we need to use evidence? • Considering risk and benefit • Decision making and using evidence • Different decisions need different evidence • How does evidence assist in decision making? • What kind of evidence is available? • Moving from anecdotal to research evidence • Evidence for effectiveness • Direct research based evidence • Indirect research based evidence • Evidence deduced from scientific knowledge • Integration of research evidence into user friendly publications • How much 'evidence' is there out there? • In summary • Key points

In this chapter we will consider:

- When do we need to use evidence?
- What types of evidence are available to help us make decisions?
- What do we do when there is limited evidence?

We will consider how to search for evidence in detail in Chapter 5.

We will discuss in greater detail how you make sense of the evidence you find in Chapter 6.

Where to start – when do we need to use evidence?

If, before you started reading this book, you thought that evidence based practice was something that concerned only the highest level decisions in health and social care, you will now be fully aware that it is something that affects all practitioners, at all levels of service provision.

In simple terms, every time you undertake a professional care activity, you make a decision about your practice. In order to make a decision, you need to ask yourself what is the evidence you need to act in this situation. This relates to all types of decisions and you need to be ready to justify your practice.

Example: if you are a physiotherapist and you regularly advise and recommend a particular type of exercise for a patient/client to follow postoperatively, you need to know the evidence base behind the exercise regime you advocate. If there is no evidence base, if it is just something that has always been advised, then this is not sufficient for an evidence based practice approach.

Example: if you are a social worker who advises young teenage single mothers about child care provision you need to know the evidence behind what has been found to be the best care for the children involved.

Example: if as a surgical nurse you promote preoperative fasting prior to surgery, you need to be able to explain and justify to your patient/client and student why this is the case and for how long this is necessary.

Considering risk and benefit

Some decisions will be more important than others. This will depend on the nature of the **risk** or **potential for harm** involved to the patient/client in undertaking or omitting the intervention and the cost involved.

Example: there is evidence that all health and social care professionals should thoroughly decontaminate their hands between every episode of patient/client contact. The evidence is very strong that hand cleansing is probably the most important strategy in infection control. This is an inexpensive task but a highly effective one which can have serious consequences if not meticulously followed. Thus, failure to follow this evidence based practice would be very difficult, if not impossible, to justify.

Example: there is now evidence about the effect of needle size on the local reaction experienced by a child following vaccination. A study was undertaken to explore the effect of the size of needle used to vaccinate young children and whether the needle size made any difference to delivery of the vaccine or local reactions experienced. Researchers in Oxford investigated the effect of needle size on effectiveness of immunogenicity and reactogenicity and identified that long, 25mm needles significantly reduced local reaction to the vaccination whilst maintaining comparable levels of immunogenicity as the shorter needle (Diggle and Deeks 2006). This is another inexpensive task, of selecting the right needle size, yet the implications of not doing so could be quite significant for the child involved and could bring bad publicity to the children's vaccination policy.

A lot of research is generated as a response to identified problems in the practice area. So, in the hand cleansing example above, the urgent need to reduce cross-infection in the clinical area led to research on the effectiveness of various ways of hand decontamination. Once the problem is identified, a research project is devised that will address the problem and the results can then be reviewed in the context of other research in the area and fed back into practice.

Whilst it might be tempting to argue that some decisions you make within your professional context are risk free, and the use of evidence is not important, this position is hard to defend. If there is good available evidence about the decision you make, you should use this in your decision making if circumstances and resources permit or there are strong reasons why this is not possible.

The greater the risk to the patient/client or likelihood of harm, the more important it is that our practice is based on evidence. However it is good practice to consider the evidence base behind all of the practice we undertake.

We know that there is no evidence to support the use of adding salt to the bath of a patient/client in order to promote wound healing. However, there is also no evidence to suggest that it is harmful. Is there anything wrong in continuing to perform outdated procedures if there is no evidence of likelihood of harm?

Decision making and using evidence

Let's look a little more closely at decision making.

Decision making is:

> A complex process involving information processing, critical thinking, evaluating evidence, applying relevant knowledge, problem solving skills, reflection and clinical judgement to select the best course of action which optimises a patient/client's health and minimises any potential harm . . .
>
> (Standing 2005 p.34)

You can see how decision making incorporates the components of evidence based practice – that is, using the best available evidence, together with professional judgement and taking consideration of patient/client preference. Standing (2005) argues that the role of the decision maker is to be professionally accountable for assessing patient/clients' needs using **appropriate sources of information** and planning interventions that address their problems. As a health and social care professional, you are making decisions about patient/client care on a day-to-day basis.

As professionals, there are a wide variety of types of decisions we make. Thompson *et al.* (2004) highlight several decision types:

- Intervention/effectiveness:
  - targeting decisions (i.e. choosing who will benefit from the intervention)
  - prevention (i.e. deciding which intervention is likely to prevent occurrence of an outcome)
  - timing of the intervention
- Referral
- Communication
- Service organisation, delivery and management
- Assessment (i.e. if an assessment is needed and what type)
- Diagnosis
- Information seeking (i.e. to either seek or not seek further information)
- Experiential, understanding or hermeneutic (i.e. relates to the interpretation of cues).

Different decisions need different evidence

Just as there are many types of decisions that you make on a daily basis, there are also many types of evidence you will use to underpin those decisions.

In general terms, you should justify the care you deliver with reference to **the most appropriate** evidence.

This will usually be from **primary research or reviews of research**. This is because research provides direct observation of the effect of interventions and care procedures on the patient/clients and clients themselves. As we have said before, ideally, this research will form the basis of policy and guidelines. However this **will not always** be the case. Sometimes research evidence will not be available. If there is no research evidence, you might draw on established scientific information and use this evidence to make reasoned deductions about what you need to know. In addition, we can draw on sociology and psychology to help us make decisions. The evidence you will be looking for will be from a varied range of sources. Sometimes you will not look to research to make your decision but would need different evidence, for example policy documents or legal precedents, or ethical rationale. Whether or not we define policy, law and ethics as 'evidence' is something that could be debated. However they certainly amount to rationale from which we draw to inform our practice. Your practice would not withstand scrutiny if you relied on outdated policy, or unlawful or unethical practice.

You are also likely to draw on professional opinion, intuition and the expertise of others when you make a decision. Remember though that these constitute the **clinical or professional judgement** component of evidence based practice and should not be confused with evidence per se.

Let's have a look at some of the decisions you are likely to be faced with in everyday practice and the **types of evidence you would need to make the right decision**.

Decision 1: My patient/client has an addiction to heroin and wants to self-discharge against the clinical judgement of staff on the ward. What should I do?

Evidence required – *relevant legal and ethical principles regarding the right of the patient/client to discharge and the duty owed to him by the health or social care professional. Local policy may also guide this decision.*

Decision 2: A member of staff has not had their vaccination for hepatitis B. As their manager how should you respond?

Evidence required – *policy for vaccination for members of staff. This policy document should be based on research evidence concerning the nature of the effectiveness of hepatitis vaccination and how it is administered.*

Decision 3: My patient/client has asked me about the use of acupuncture as a pain-relieving agent. What evidence would you need to be able to discuss this with the patient/client?

Evidence required – *to answer any questions about the effectiveness of an intervention, you would need to find research – ideally in the form of randomised controlled trials that have looked specifically at the issue in question (we will discuss what randomised controlled trials are and why they are needed later on).*

Decision 4: A client seeks advice on smoking cessation. How should you advise him or her?

Evidence required – *there is a wealth of research based evidence on smoking cessation which can be accessed according to the situation of the client. A systematic review may provide a summary of the information you need.*

Decision 5: A client asks you for advice on preventing post-surgery complications.

Evidence required – *evidence regarding effectiveness of preventing postoperative interventions will come from randomised controlled trials.*

Decision 6: A client with depression wants to have greater access to his children.

Evidence required – *you will need to explore his rights as a father from a legal perspective and the implications of his depression on his ability to care for his children which may come from qualitative research about the experiences of those with depression coping with parenthood.*

It is important to remember that the main point is to use the most appropriate form of evidence to address what you need to find out. This might be research evidence, policy, or legal or ethical principles. There will often be policies and guidelines you can draw on. Remember as well that it is important to identify a question that captures what you need to find out. When you seek to use evidence in your professional practice, this is sometimes referred to as practising in an 'evidence informed way'. In order to do this, the first thing you need to do is define a question that identifies what you need to know. This is important because unless you have a focussed question, you will not be able to work out how to find the answer and you will be swamped with information. You are therefore likely to end up more confused than when you started! We will discuss this in more detail in Chapter 5.

How does evidence assist in decision making?

We have already mentioned that evidence alone is not enough to make a good decision if you are practising in an evidence informed way. You need to exercise **your own professional judgement** and consider the **preferences of the**

patient/client. Standing (2008) argues that there are also likely to be many other factors that you consider when making a clinical decision and it will depend on the complexity of the decision and the time available. If you have sufficient time available to you and the appropriate resources, you will be able to make a considered and rational decision, fully informed by relevant evidence. If you have less time and there is a moment of crisis, your decision is likely to be more reactionary. This is where the use of policy and guidelines are useful as they provide guidance in a situation where you need to make a quick decision.

Standing (2008) had put this in a diagrammatic form. See Figure 3.1.

What kind of evidence is available?

There are many different kinds of evidence that will assist your decision making:

- Research that is directly relevant to your patient/client
- Research that has been carried out on different patient/client groups
- Basic scientific/social scientific research which we use to make deductions about patient/client care.

Moving from anecdotal to research evidence

As we have said before, evidence comes in many forms. There is both strong and weak evidence and we will discuss this in greater detail in Chapter 6. However, if you are asked to underpin your practice with evidence, you need to know exactly what you mean by this. You are probably familiar with the term anecdotal evidence. This is generally a weaker form of evidence.

Anecdotal evidence

Example: Imagine you are trying to train your dog. He is not an easy dog to train – he is somewhat feisty and pulls on the lead. You try out a few choker collars which pull tighter around his neck when he pulls and relaxes when he walks nicely to heel. You aim to see which one he responds to the best. You find one that seems to be a good fit and deters him from pulling on the lead. Here you have some evidence about which choker lead works best – at

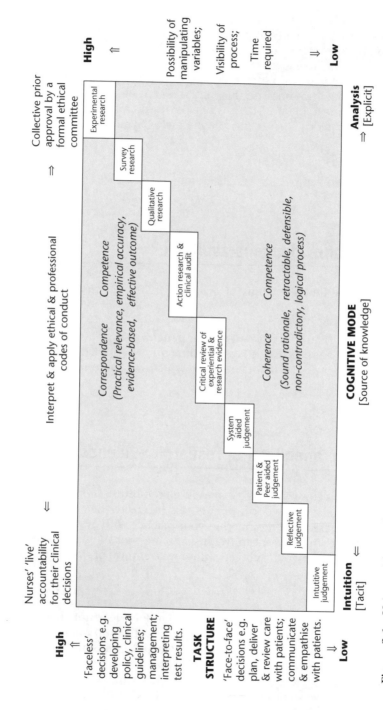

Figure 3.1 Using evidence, Standing 2008.

least for you and your dog. This is anecdotal evidence and is the type of evidence that people have gathered and used over the generations. Indeed a lot of health and social and social care has been based on anecdotal evidence in the absence of harder evidence being available.

Now imagine that you have hundreds of dogs at a Guide Dog training centre and you need to know which lead works the best. **Here the stakes are higher for many reasons:**

- The effective training of the dogs is even more important because of the role they are to perform.
- The cost of the lead must be multiplied by the number of dogs so there is a big cost implication.
- The time taken to train the dog also has cost implications.

If you were a recipient of a guide dog or a donator to the charitable organisation Guide Dogs for the Blind, you would want to know that the best lead was being used to train the dogs. In this instance, the anecdotal evidence gained from the experience of one person attempting to train his dog would not seem sufficient. You would want more robust evidence upon which to base your choice of dog lead.

This scenario can be transferred to health and social care settings in which the stakes are high. There are limited resources and patient/clients have an expectation and a right to receive the optimum care. **We cannot afford to get it wrong.** Anecdotal evidence – or trial and error – is clearly not enough. We cannot afford to base practice on insubstantial evidence which does not stand up to scrutiny.

In health and social care, **anecdotal evidence** can be:

- Using something you've tried before that worked
- Your colleague or practice assessor/mentor who says 'we've always done it like this'
- Discussion papers, opinion articles or editorials
- Expert opinion (consultants, specialist practitioners, other professionals, although their opinion is very likely to be informed by evidence – but do not make this assumption!).

In principle, you should be aware that the quality of evidence provided by anecdotal information – even if it is based on expert opinion – is generally weaker than that which is provided by empirical study. Remember that if you do not ask for the evidence that lies behind the advice you are given, you might be practising using anecdotal evidence only and your practice would not stand up to scrutiny. However, published material that does not report research findings can still be useful. This is why it is important to determine what evidence you need in the first instance. Anecdotal information can be useful in the following ways:

- It can contribute to your professional judgement.
- It can be used to set the context/give background information.
- It can be used to identify what common practice is in the light of little other evidence.
- It might be used to address the research question directly if there is minimal research on the topic.
- It might also be used directly to address the research question e.g. if you are specifically looking at how the media portrays the role of the occupational therapist, then media cuttings will be of utmost relevance to your review.

In the same way as the Guide Dog trainer needs good evidence about the effectiveness of the different dog leads available, so does the health and social care provider needs good evidence about the effectiveness of the care they deliver. With the availability of systematic and rigorous research studies, we now have more robust evidence upon which to base our practice.

Research based evidence

So if we need to move away from anecdotal evidence, what do we move towards?

The **simple answer** is that usually, evidence from **research studies** will provide stronger evidence upon which to build our practice. Evidence provided by a **review of many studies** will make even stronger evidence.

Empirical evidence is that which is obtained directly from scientific observation or experimenting/research in practice. This can be research that relates directly to our practice, research that is indirectly related to our practice and /or deductions made from scientific knowledge.

What is important is that we ensure that we use the **right evidence** to underpin practice. Think back to the examples given earlier – different types of evidence were required for each decision in question. When you are looking for evidence on your topic, 'one size' really does not fit all. If anyone tells you that you *'always need research evidence'* to answer your question they will be wrong – you need the most relevant information that will answer your question. The evidence you need might come from another source. Furthermore, you might hear someone saying that randomised controlled trials (RCTs) are the 'gold standard' of evidence that you need. This is often not the case as RCTs only help you if you are looking at whether a treatment or care is effective. If you are not looking at effectiveness, then RCTs will not be the 'gold standard' evidence for your question.

Example: To illustrate this, let's think about a product that came onto the market in 2008, in the light of the smoking ban that exists now in many countries, which is the electric cigarette. Apparently, it is perfectly legal to smoke these cigarettes in public areas where conventional cigarettes would be banned. The manufacturers claim that although there are no or minimal known health and social risks, the product can be used to enhance smoking cessation strategies because they deliver a reduced amount of nicotine, mimicking the effects of conventional cigarettes.

A friend of yours asks you about these electric cigarettes. You promise that you will find some information/evidence about them and endeavour to do so. Where would you start?

First of all, as we have already discussed, you would need to clarify exactly what your friend wants to know. What question is (s)he asking of you? Is (s)he concerned about the usefulness of electric cigarettes in assisting with smoking cessation? Or is (s)he concerned with the health and social effects of the cigarettes? Or is (s)he mostly concerned to find out whether the electric cigarettes are really as pleasurable as the advertisements suggest. If you do not identify exactly what your friend wants to know you will not be able to find the appropriate evidence to advise him or her in a meaningful way. You might find out about the health and social risks of these cigarettes whilst what (s)he really wanted to know is about their role in smoking cessation. The information you do find might give some reference to smoking cessation, but given that this was not what you were looking for, this evidence is likely to be of limited usefulness. Thus the message is clear – you need to know what evidence you are looking for before you begin!

Once you have established this, you need to identify what sort of evidence you need. The evidence you need will depend on the type of question you are asking. If you are looking for evidence about the effectiveness or safety of electric cigarettes as a smoking cessation intervention, this evidence will not be the same as that you would look for if you were looking for evidence about the pleasure effect of electric cigarettes. Organisations such as the World Health Organization (WHO) and the anti-smoking charity ASH will often offer counter-arguments for such innovations.

If you can only find information about claims of the effectiveness of electric cigarettes in advertisements on the website of the manufacturers, or that they had only carried out animal and not human trials on safety how strong would you think this evidence would be?

Answer: This is likely to be anecdotal evidence only or it may be biased in its approach.

Evidence for effectiveness

If you need to know about the effectiveness of the electric cigarettes, the only way to really tell if something is effective is to find a randomised controlled trial (RCT). This is because in an RCT there is a control group who do not receive the intervention in question who act as a direct comparison. Therefore in this case, RCTs are the 'gold standard' of evidence you are looking for. If the manufacturers are telling you that their product is effective, but you cannot find an RCT to back this up, then you should be wary of that claim! We will discuss this further in the next chapter.

Evidence about an experience is different from evidence about effectiveness.

If you are looking for evidence about the pleasure aspect of smoking electric cigarettes, an RCT is unlikely to help you, unless you found one that compared the pleasure obtained from smoking the electric cigarette with another type of cigarette. Instead, you could look for research reports that explore the person's experience. This is likely to be through asking them about it. If you find a lot of general information or evidence but cannot find any evidence that looks specifically at this aspect, then you would have to tell your friend that you could not find any relevant evidence. Therefore, you need to think carefully about what sort of evidence you need to answer specific questions that arise that require evidence.

Example: you are concerned about infection in your unit and want to find out about how compliant staff are with hand-washing/hand-rubbing policies. What type of evidence would you look for? Imagine you found a questionnaire study that had asked staff at the end of every shift whether they always follow infection control procedures. What answers are they likely to give? Do you think these would reflect what they *actually* do? How strong would that evidence be?

What type of evidence would you be looking for that would really tell you about staff adherence to infection control policy?

Clearly the answer is to find studies (**observational**) that have seen if staff washed their hands or not in the everyday context. Any evidence that falls short of this approach would not be very strong. Thus for this question, the very best type of evidence would be observational studies.

There are many forms of evidence – some of which will be stronger than others. When we are thinking about evidence based practice, we need to ensure that we use the strongest possible evidence to support our practice. If we do not seek out strong evidence, we risk being criticised for not using up-to-date, robust evidence. Remember that the nature of evidence in health and social care changes very quickly and what was considered good evidence at one time can become quickly outdated. However you must also remember that nothing is perfect and you may not always be able to find strong evidence. You should aim to base your practice on the best available evidence you can find.

Direct research based evidence

Direct research based evidence is evidence that **relates directly** to the health and social care practice situation you are involved with.

In an ideal world, there would be direct evidence to underpin the care you deliver and this evidence would be based on direct observations or studies of people who are similar to those you look after. Also in an ideal world, you would find that the evidence that exists relates directly to your clinical or professional setting so that you can be as sure as possible that it applies to your patient or client.

An example would be that of hand cleansing. The process of hand cleansing is the same whichever patient/clients you work with, except of course that some patient/clients are under additional infection control precautions. Research evidence relating to hand cleansing will be relevant to your practice irrespective of where and when it was undertaken, although you still need to assess the quality of the research undertaken which we will look at later in this book.

A further example of direct evidence would be the impact of shift work on the quality of care. Shift work is an integral component of all practice areas where patient/clients require 24-hour care. Thus any research which explores quality of care provision and its relationship to shift work is likely to be directly relevant to all disciplines.

However, more often than not, you will come across evidence that does not relate directly to your patient/client or client group or the exact situation you encounter. This evidence can still be useful to you. We will refer to this as **indirect research based evidence**.

Indirect research based evidence

 Indirect research based evidence is evidence that does not relate specifically to your practice but is none the less relevant to your practice. The research might have been carried out on a different group of patients or clients or in a different country, so its relevance and application to your setting might be different.

Example: An example of the use and relevance of indirect evidence could be research about how information giving reduces anxiety. Let's say that you come across some research that was undertaken with patient/clients in an oncology ward. You are working in general surgery. This evidence will be less directly relevant to your patient/clients and you need to determine the extent to which the research is relevant to you. We will discuss ways of assessing the quality of the evidence further on in this book but for now it is important to note that you are likely to have to make a judgement about the applicability of the evidence you encounter to your professional practice. This is the 'clinical/professional judgement' component of evidence based practice we referred to in Chapter 1. However this research will be relevant to you in some way. This is why we refer to it as indirect evidence.

Example: Imagine you are working with deprived children in an inner city from a particular cultural group. There is research evidence about the most effective way to promote uptake of day care provision that has been undertaken with a different cultural group but nothing that relates to the particular group of children you are working with. Again, this is where your clinical or professional judgement comes into play. You might find that this is the best available evidence and you need to determine how relevant it is to the group of children you are working with.

Example: Another example of indirect evidence is the use of antiseptic skin washing prior to surgery. Whilst there is evidence to suggest that use of a skin wash does reduce the amount of surface bacteria on the skin, there is, to date, no available evidence that this reduced skin bacterial count leads to reduced rates of infection following surgery. There have been some clinical trials which have compared the rates of infection in patient/clients who used an antiseptic skin wash and those who did not and none of the trials found any benefit, or reduced rate of infection in those who applied the antiseptic skin wash. However you might argue that it still seems logical to require all patient/clients to use the skin wash prior to surgery, given that there is some scientific or theoretical evidence that skin bacterial counts will be reduced. Thus, patient/clients are commonly advised to use the antiseptic skin wash prior to surgery, but we are unable to give a rationale other than use of the antiseptic reduces skin bacteria (but not necessarily postoperative infection rates).

Given this information, do you feel that use of antiseptic skin washing prior to surgery fits into an evidence based approach? Would you choose to wash with the solution or not?

You are probably thinking by now that much of the evidence you use in your clinical practice is indirect evidence – that is, even if it was obtained through direct observation or experiments on patient or clients, its focus was not on the practice setting you are working in and therefore the evidence does not apply to your practice directly and you have to make a judgement about its relevance to your practice area. You will find that this is often the case.

Evidence deduced from scientific knowledge

Evidence deduced from scientific knowledge is where you take principles from the sciences and apply them to the practice setting.

It might be that you find that there is no direct or indirect research evidence that is relevant to the area you are searching for information about. It will often be the case that there is not sufficient direct or indirect research evidence available to you about the specific question you are investigating.

Does this mean that you cannot practice evidence based practice? The answer is you can still find evidence to underpin your practice, even if it is not immediately obvious what information might be relevant to you.

However, to do so, it will be necessary to look further afield for sources that might provide you with an evidence base for your practice. This is because professional practice encompasses a very wide range of activities and will therefore draw on a wide range of sources of evidence to justify practice.

Your practice can be underpinned by **evidence which is deduced from scientific knowledge rather than from observation on patient or clients themselves.**

Evidence deduced from scientific knowledge is evidence which is obtained from scientific and social scientific explanations about how things work, but which have not been tested or observed scientifically (empirically) with patient or clients in the practice setting. By scientific knowledge we mean from the hard sciences, such as biology, physiology and also from social sciences such as sociology and psychology.

Sciences from which we might draw evidence include: physiology and patho-physiology, medicine (many branches), pharmacology, sociology, immunology, dietetics, radiology, epidemiology, cytology, microbiology, gerontology, anatomy, psychiatry, psychology, podiatry.

Example: Let's take the example information giving about alcohol intake for pregnant women. We know that alcohol intake during pregnancy is likely to lead to low birth weight babies. We also know that low birth weight babies are also more likely to spend time in the intensive care unit. We can deduce from this that alcohol consumption during pregnancy is likely to lead to increased risk of admission to intensive care for the new born child, however unless we find out about the alcohol consumption of mothers of babies in intensive care we cannot say for certain that alcohol consumption during pregnancy increases the chances of intensive care admission for the baby. For this, we would need empirical evidence because you are testing or scientifically observing what actually happens in practice.

Example: Another example of evidence that is deduced from scientific knowledge would be that of taking patient/clients' physiological observations. We know from our understanding of physiology that taking the patient/client's vital signs – temperature, pulse and blood pressure – will give an indication of the condition of the patient/client. We also know that low blood pressure readings are indicative of haemorrhage. There is, therefore, a physiological rationale for taking a patient/client's blood pressure following surgery. Yet in order to really know how effective this practice is in the prevention and management of haemorrhage we would need to observe the effectiveness of this in practice. Interestingly, Zeitz and McCutcheon (2003) undertook a literature search for the empirical rationale for the frequent blood pressure measurement following surgery. They found that despite the physiological rational for blood pressure monitoring, there was an absence of direct evidence to support frequent blood pressure measurement.

Another **example** of evidence which is drawn from a wider body of research is the practice of laying out a patient/client shortly after death has occurred. Philpin (2002) suggests that those very serious about evidence based practice would oppose this practice, arguing that it is a ritual for which there is no scientific rationale. However if we look to the wider psychological and sociological literature surrounding dignity, grief and coping with death of a loved one, we are likely to find justification and evidence to support this activity. If, on the other hand, no justification could be found in the psychological or sociological literature as a rationale for the 'ritual' of laying out a person after death has occurred, or it was found that this 'ritual' was the cause of further distress, there would be evidence against it.

All our professions rely on knowledge from many different disciplines, including sociology, psychology, pharmacology to name but a few.

What other specialist disciplines predominantly inform your professional practices?

You are likely to find that your own area of practice is informed by a wide variety of disciplines and that research from within these disciplines will be relevant to your practice. You will use these to develop an understanding of the evidence base behind many of the activities you undertake. You might therefore need to think quite broadly to find evidence to justify your practice.

Integration of research evidence into user friendly publications

Often you will find that you do not find the 'raw' data from the research but instead you find publications which have used the evidence from direct and indirect research. Examples of such publications are:

- Government or professional organisations' policy, reports, guidance or standards
- Care pathways or protocols
- Results from audits
- Reports from international, national or local organisations
- Information from trusted websites
- Patient/client information leaflets
- Information leaflets/letters from manufacturers regarding products
- Textbooks.

Can you identify areas of your own practice that may have an evidence base you can use?

You can find out this by:

- Accessing a professional journal that focusses on your profession
- Using professional associations' websites
- Attending conferences accessing conference presentations online if unable to attend

- Identifying areas in your own practice where you are unsure of your practice or there is inconsistency between practitioners
- Reflecting on your practice out loud (this often highlights areas where you are unable to provide a rationale or the rationale is weak)
- Having discussions on your practice with colleagues or specialists
- Networking – visiting or making contact with other specialists in your field and sharing how you practise
- Asking students or new staff to your area if they observe any unfamiliar practices or things that conflict with what they have learnt previously.

How much 'evidence' is there out there?

You will not always find direct or indirect research information on your topic – either a literature review or individual piece of research.

Imagine a line where traditional practices and ritual were at one end and a fully evidence based approach was at the other.

ritualistic practice   evidence based practice

◄───►

You would probably like to think that the majority of health and social care procedures fall at the evidence based end of the continuum. However, unfortunately it is not as straightforward as this. In 1992, in a controversial statement, Smith (1991) argued that around only 10–20% of medical interventions had evidence that they provided a positive effect on patient/client health. This assertion caused much outcry and since then medical practitioners have taken up the challenge to disprove this claim (Ellis *et al.* 1995; Gill *et al.* 1996) and to demonstrate that much more of their practice is based on evidence. We have not yet found any such studies of other professional groups, so the extent to which practice within health and social care is based on evidence of effectiveness is unknown.

No evidence at all?

Sometimes you may not find any research based information, or you might not be in a position to identify the best possible evidence. In this case you will rely on weaker sources, such as experience, advice from colleagues but you should be aware that these provide a weaker source of evidence. You should always try to avoid relying on unknown sources of information, such as those you might come across on the internet.

If you think about your own everyday practice, how much do you think should or can be based on actual high quality evidence?

Evidence to look for

- **Systematic literature reviews** – probably the most important single source of evidence, we will explain why after this section.
- **Research papers** – but one paper alone is generally not enough. Primary research is most often published in journals and you will tend to find the most up-to-date resources on your topic in journal articles rather than in textbooks. This is because the subject matter of most textbooks tends to be quite broad and is quickly out of date. Also remember that the research must be relevant to the research question you need to address. If you find one research paper on a topic, search for another and see how the results compare.
- **Policy documents** – see if these are based on research evidence.
- **Legal and ethical guidance.**

Evidence to beware of

- **Evidence obtained through broad use of search engines.** Beware of sources retrieved through random **search engine** searches such as **GOOGLE**. The ability to search is limited and so the information you find may be too broad and of poor quality. Whilst it might throw up some genuinely interesting and useful information or even allow you to access an article you have been looking for, it is difficult to find this information in the midst of the less useful information that you will come across. This is because search engines are broad and search for everything on the topic entered. Clearly not everything entered on the internet on your topic will be of high quality. There is nobody to police the internet and websites can be created by anyone. Whilst this freedom of expression has many positive attributes, it does mean that you have to be discerning when you search using search engines.
- **Unknown websites.** Websites can be useful. We will discuss this in Chapter 6. However, it is vital that you assess the sources upon which the website is based.
- **Textbooks.** Textbooks are useful sources of general information but tend to provide a general introduction to a subject (such as the purpose of this book) rather than providing in-depth evidence. Therefore whether you use textbooks or not depends on what you need to find out and how recently the textbook was written.
- **One single piece of non-research based evidence that makes a claim about practice.** This might be an opinion piece found in a professional journal. We will consider how to judge the quality of the evidence that you

find in Chapter 6 but the point we would like to make here is that one piece of literature, even research, is rarely enough for you to base your practice on.

In relation to our previous example about the electronic cigarette your friend may not be satisfied with the quality or quantity of the evidence you found. *'So you have found one questionnaire study, undertaken in a bar in south London to convince me that these electric cigarettes are useful to assist people in quitting smoking?? I need some stronger evidence!'*

In summary

Every time you make a decision you need to consider the evidence base you can draw on to make the decision. Asking your colleague or practice assessor/ mentor is not enough! Research based evidence should normally be drawn on in the first instance and this may be linked directly or less directly to your area of practice. If no research evidence is available, then you will draw on weaker evidence. It is important to recognise how strong the evidence is that you draw upon as this reflects how much confidence you can have in the evidence you use.

Key points

1 Every time you make a decision, you need to consider what evidence you need to base your decision upon.
2 There are many different types of decision and many different types of evidence to use.
3 You will **normally** use research evidence in the first instance.
4 At other times you will need a different rationale – for example ethical principles or legal guidance.
5 Some research will be directly relevant to your question, other research will be less directly relevant.
6 You might also use physiological, psychological, sociological, pharmaco- logical evidence.
7 Policy and guidelines should be based on research evidence.
8 Use anecdotal evidence as a last resort.

4

What are the different types of research? How do these different types of evidence help us answer different questions?

Reviews of quantitative or qualitative research • Why are reviews so useful? • Putting the evidence into context • Helping to shed new light • How can I recognise a literature review when I see one? • What different types of literature reviews are there? • The systematic review • Literature reviews (using less detailed approaches) • Quantitative research • Quasi experiments • Cohort studies and case control studies • Questionnaire/surveys/cross-sectional studies • Sampling in quantitative research • Qualitative studies • Which type of research is best? • I have read about the term 'hierarchy of evidence'. What does it mean? • What about using secondary sources? • Professional and clinical guidance • Non-research based evidence • In summary • Key points

In the previous chapter, we provided an overview of the different kinds of evidence that are available to assist you with using an evidence based approach to your practice. In this chapter we will consider:

- The different types of research and other evidence that you might find.
- How the question you want answering influences the type of evidence you look for.

We acknowledge that evidence based practice does not necessarily mean that you will always be using research evidence – but this is often the case. Therefore, given that research can be hard to understand, we have devoted this chapter to summarising what types of research evidence you are likely to encounter.

Brainstorm research methods have you heard of.

The research methods outlined below are just some of the methods that you might encounter. It is important that you are familiar with the different approaches to research design so that you can judge the relevance and quality of it. We will discuss this in greater detail in Chapter 6.

Research evidence can be classified as follows:

- **Reviews** of either qualitative or quantitative research
- **Quantitative research**
  - **experimental methods** (where an intervention is given to one group and not to another and the outcomes observed), for example, randomised controlled trials (RCTs)
  - **non-experimental methods** (where no intervention is given and populations are observed and compared to a control group), for example, cohort and case controlled studies, cross-sectional studies, questionnaires/surveys
- **Qualitative research**
  - grounded theory
  - phenomenology
  - ethnography
  - action research
- **Guidelines and policy** (which are based on research evidence).

Reviews of quantitative or qualitative research (sometimes known as systematic reviews or literature reviews)

A review is a collection of research papers on a specified topic. A systematic review is a very detailed review on a topic. A literature review usually refers to a review that is less systematic. We will discuss these terms in more detail as we go on.

Why are reviews so useful?

Literature reviews are important because they seek to:

- Summarise the literature that is available on any one topic
- Prevent one 'high profile' piece of information having too much influence
- Present an analysis of the available literature so that the reader does not have to access each individual research report included in the review.

It often seems to be the case that a piece of research is published one month which contradicts the findings of a piece of research published the month before. For example, one week we are told that alcohol has certain health benefits, the next week we are told that it is harmful. There is often then an outcry – people are confused by the differing messages conveyed and wonder why the results can vary so much. This can be due to:

- The media portrayal of the research in which a complex set of results is reduced to a simplified message.
- There are many aspects of health; alcohol might have a positive effect on one aspect and a damaging effect on another.
- The fact that any one individual piece of research, or health and social care information, is like just one part of a large jigsaw. It does not represent the whole picture – it represents merely a section of that picture and needs to be set in the context of other information.

An individual piece of health and social care information, taken in isolation, does not necessarily help the reader to achieve a better understanding of the bigger picture towards which the information contributes. There are many reasons for this:

- The research might have been undertaken in a specific area of practice or

with a specific group of people, or sample, and is not generalisable (or applicable) to other areas.
- There might be flaws in the research design which affect its overall useful-ness. Therefore when you read a report that seems to conflict with a report you read the previous week, it is important to consider the merits of each individual report and to remember that each single piece of research should not be viewed in isolation.

Let's go into a little more detail as to why this is. One isolated piece of literature can be misleading. Take the story of the measles, mumps and rubella (MMR) vaccine. In 1998, Professor Wakefield and colleagues published an article in the *Lancet* suggesting that there was a possibility of a link between the MMR vaccination, autism and bowel disorders. This article was based on a small case study of twelve children, who had attended Wakefield's hospital, who had the conditions above and who had also had the vaccin-ation. Wakefield stated that there were possible environmental triggers to the development of autism in these children, but without controls this was very uncertain.

The paper published by Wakefield provided one piece of the jigsaw. At that time, there were no other data surrounding any potential link between autism and bowel disease. However, as time went on, many further studies were undertaken. No further studies confirmed any evidence of a link. It is easy to identify from the basic facts presented in the original paper that the evi-dence presented is not strong. However, seen in isolation, this report sparked alarm in both media and medical circles alike.

Putting the evidence into context

This is why literature reviews are so important in health and social care because they enable the reader to view each piece of research within the con-text of others. Take, for example, Linus Pauling (1986), the world accredited scientist, who wrote a book entitled *How to live longer and feel better*, in which he quoted from a selection of articles that supported his opinion that vitamin C contains properties that are effective against the common cold. This book makes an interesting and convincing read. However, the arguments presented in the book were challenged some years later by Professor Knipschild (1994), who undertook a systematic review of all of the evidence surrounding the effectiveness of vitamin C and came to very different conclusions. He argued that Pauling had not looked systematically at all the research and had selected only articles that supported his view whilst apparently ignoring those that did not. This is why, when you read a report by an expert in a particular area, you should remember that this report represents just an expert view which might not be substantiated by evidence. This is why expert opinion is generally not considered to be a strong form of evidence.

Helping to shed new light

The MMR controversy provides one clear example as to why it is important to review all the evidence together and how one piece of information can give a misleading picture. Without the comprehensive review of the literature which followed Wakefield's paper, the concerns expressed in his initial paper could not have been refuted. In a recent Cochrane review (Parsons *et al.* 2008), the role of a drug used to facilitate weight loss was reviewed. It had been previously thought that the use of drugs played only a minor role in weight loss facilitation programmes. On reviewing the available literature in a systematic way, the role of these drugs was found to be larger than had been thought.

How can I recognise a literature review when I see one?

This is an important question. A literature review will be written up in the same manner as a research article; it should have:

- A clear research/review question
- Aims and objectives
- A methods section outlining how the review was undertaken.

You might find a discussion article which has included various references and you wonder if this is a literature review. You may also find an article explaining about a particular topic and wonder if this is a literature review. In short it probably is not.

If the information you find does not contain a research question, aims and objectives and a methods section, then it is unlikely to be a literature review.

What different types of literature reviews are there?

You are likely to come across different types of literature reviews and it is useful to be able to recognise the types of reviews that exist.

It is important that all reviews are approached in a systematic manner so that all the available information is incorporated into the review. You would not feel very confident reading a review which had omitted a lot of relevant information. However, when you read literature reviews, you will discover that some are undertaken in more detail than others. The most detailed type of literature review is often referred to as a **systematic review.**

The systematic review

A systematic review aims to identify and track down all the available literature on a topic with clear explanations of the approach taken (methodology). Systematic literature reviews are referred to as original empirical research as they review primary data, which can be either quantitative or qualitative. Systematic reviews which have a detailed research methodology should be regarded as a strong form of evidence when they are identified as relevant to a literature review question.

Systematic reviews were first defined as 'concise summaries of the best available evidence that address sharply defined clinical questions' (Mulrow *et al.* 1997 p.389).

The most well known method for conducting a systematic review is produced by the **Cochrane Collaboration.** The Cochrane Collaboration was established in 1993 and is a large international organisation whose purpose is to provide independent systematically produced reviews about the effectiveness of health and social care interventions. See the Cochrane website where you can browse by topic for reviews and they have a plain English summary to help you understand complex jargon.

Cochrane Library available at http://www.cochrane.org/reviews/

The NHS National Library for Health also provides links to several other evidence based review sites available at http://www.library.nhs.uk/Default. http://www.cochrane.org/reviews/en/topics/index.html

A systematic review undertaken in the detail required by the Cochrane

Collaboration is usually considered to be the most detailed and robust form of review that exists. For example, in the United Kingdom they are used in the formulation of guidelines for the National Institute for Health and Clinical Excellence (NICE) available at http://www.nice.org.uk/ whose recommendations for clinical practice are based on the best available evidence.

The main features of a systematic review are that the reviewers

- Follow *strict guidelines* to ensure that the review is systematic
- Use clear and thorough methods to identify and critically appraise relevant studies in order to answer a *predefined question*
- Leave no stone unturned in the search for relevant literature, and do not regard the process complete until the search is exhausted
- Search for articles that have not been published or not yet accepted for publication. The reason for this is that there is evidence that results are more likely to be published if they show the benefit of an intervention than those which do not (using only published data could bias the result of the review)
- Develop *inclusion and exclusion criteria* in order to assess which information should be included in the review to ensure that only those papers that are relevant to the question(s) are included
- *Critique* (or judge) the selected papers according to predetermined criteria in order to assess the quality of the research identified. Studies that do not meet the inclusion criteria are excluded from the review. This is to ensure that only high quality papers that are relevant to the literature review question are included. The results of research that has been poorly carried out are likely to be less reliable and may bias the findings of the review
- Finally *combine* the findings of all the papers that are used using a systematic approach. This enables new insights to be drawn from the summary of the papers that was not available before.

Look on one of the sites for systematic reviews and find a topic relevant to your own professional practice that has been reviewed.

An example of a systematic review is the review carried out by Demicheli *et al.* (2006) who examined the evidence regarding a link between autism, bowel disease and the measles, mumps and rubella (MMR) vaccination. Following a comprehensive and rigorous review of the evidence in this systematic review, the authors were able to declare that they found no evidence of a link between autism, bowel disease and MMR vaccine.

The methods of undertaking a systematic review are time consuming and usually require the involvement of a team of experienced researchers over a period of time.

Literature reviews (using less detailed approaches)

A literature review can be approached in a systematic manner even if the detail required by the Cochrane Collaboration is not attained. Whilst the term 'systematic review' is often used to refer to reviews undertaken according to the Cochrane Collaboration method of reviewing, it is sometimes referred to as a review of the literature using a systematic approach, but which is less rigorous and detailed than the methods described above. There can therefore be some confusion concerning the meaning of a systematic review.

You may also come across 'literature reviews' which are undertaken with no defined method or systematic approach. These are sometimes referred to as narrative reviews. A narrative review might be no more than a biased collection of research papers and other information about a given topic.

They generally:

- Have no focussed research question
- Have no focussed searching strategy
- Have no clear method of appraisal or synthesis of literature
- Are not easily repeatable.

Consequently, the conclusions drawn are likely to be inaccurate. You should be cautious of these narrative reviews as they are likely to miss out some information. These or narrative 'traditional' reviews have a number of biases. There is normally the personal bias of the author/s, no clear methodology, a bias in the selection of included material and conclusions which cannot be easily verified and may be misleading.

As a health and social care professional you cannot be expected to read, evaluate, assimilate and apply all the information on any one topic even if you could find it in the first place! Therefore, if you come across a literature review that has been undertaken on the topic on which you are seeking evidence, consider this a lucky find indeed. It is as if you have unearthed the whole jigsaw rather than just one or two pieces of it.

Quantitative research

Quantitative research (sometimes called positivist research) normally refers to studies which use methods of data collection that involve *the use of numbers*.

- Quantitative research is appropriate only for when data can be collected numerically – for example the **number** of 'symptom-free years' experienced by a patient/client.

- Data are analysed using statistical tests.
- The studies tend to involve many participants and the findings can be applied in other contexts.
- Traditionally there is no involvement between the researcher and participant.

For example, quantitative **experimental** methods can be used to measure the effectiveness of an intervention (for example, smoking cessation interventions). In this case, quantitative methods could be used to compare how many people give up smoking in the intervention group and in the non-intervention group. This would be measured numerically, in months and years. The important thing here is that the experimenter controls who has what intervention. Hence we call it an experiment.

Quantitative research methods can also be used for **non-experimental** research designs, such as questionnaire/surveys in which participants respond to questions. Their responses can then be counted numerically – for example 30% of those who responded to the survey had done X.

In principle quantitative research is generally undertaken when you are looking to measure something and that something is suitable for numerical measurement. Let's look in more detail at some of the quantitative research designs that you are likely to encounter.

Randomised controlled trials (RCTs) are a form of clinical trial, or scientific procedure used to determine the *effectiveness* of a treatment or medicine.

RCTs are useful when . . . you are looking to find out **whether a treatment or intervention is effective**. In this case, you should search for RCTs in the first instance. If you find some RCTs, then you probably have good evidence about the effectiveness of your treatment or intervention. If you do not find any RCTs then you cannot answer your question regarding whether the intervention is effective.

Randomised controlled trials are the best way (and many people would say the only way) to determine whether a treatment or intervention is effective or not. They can be used to test out the effectiveness of many care or treatment options where it is permissible to randomly divide the sample group and monitor the outcome. It is often commented that RCTs are not used sufficiently within health and social care and hence we do not know enough about the effectiveness of interventions.

- They are widely considered to be the most thorough ('gold standard') form of evidence when we are considering whether a treatment or intervention is effective.

- In an RCT, participants are allocated by random allocation into two or more groups.
- An intervention is then given to one of the groups and not given to the other (control) group; the outcome of the two groups is then compared.
- If it is not possible to randomise participants in a research study and expose one group to a particular procedure (e.g. for ethical reasons) then it is not possible to carry out an RCT.

How does randomisation work?

Participants are allocated into the different treatment groups of the trial at **random**. This is like the tossing of a coin. This ensures that participants are allocated into the different groups by chance rather than by the preference of the patient/client or researcher. It is very important that neither the participant nor the researcher has any control over the group to which a participant is allocated.

Why is randomisation important?

Randomisation is important because the researcher is looking for differences between the treatment group and the control group. If the groups are random, then any differences in outcome are likely to be due to the intervention. This can only be determined if the different groups, which are commonly referred to as arms, of the trial are essentially equal in all respects except for the treatment given. The researcher is looking for differences between the different groups of the trial that can be attributed to the intervention (such as symptoms, mobility, pain, improvements).

Do the groups in an RCT have similar characteristics after randomisation?

The randomisation process normally results in the creation of equal groups. If it is particularly important that participants with specific characteristics are equally represented in both groups (for example, those in certain age groups or those with young children might have different lifestyle habits from those without children and you might want an equal number of these participants in each group) then a further form of randomisation can be used. This is an additional statistical process that assists in ensuring that the groups are equal in respect of certain predefined criteria that are relevant for the research, and is called stratification or minimisation.

Why can't participants choose which group they want to go into?

Randomisation is important because if the research participants were allowed to choose which group of the RCT they wanted to enter, it is very likely that one particular treatment group would be more popular than another. Then the trial could not be carried out. Also the different groups in the trial would not be equal. Let's say that researchers wanted to explore a new drug for helping people to lose weight. They need to allocate participants by random assignment into one of two treatment or control groups of the trial. If either the researcher or participant had been allowed to choose who should go in each group, those more committed to the lifestyle change might have chosen the arm of the trial with the intervention and those who were less committed might have chosen the arm of the trial with the standard care or dummy tablet (placebo). The two treatment groups of the trial would then not be equal. It would then not be possible to determine whether the differences in outcomes observed between the different treatment or control groups of the trial were due to the new drug or whether they were due to the differences in the characteristics of the participants who had self selected into one group or another.

How does an RCT work?

Once each treatment group in the trial has been randomly allocated, the groups are considered to be equal, and the intervention treatment is given to group one. The second group receives either the standard treatment (or no treatment or placebo, depending on the individual study design). The groups are then observed and the differences between the groups in terms of weight loss are monitored. Given that the two groups of participants were randomly allocated and hence can be considered to be 'equal', any difference in between the groups can be attributed to the effect of the drug.

The non-intervention group may be:

- **A control group** who receive the established standard treatment (while another group receive the new intervention)
- **A placebo group** who receive a dummy drug or sham treatment, but the important thing is that the participants do not know this! A placebo group is however only ethical if non-treatment is not thought to be harmful to participants – let's say if there was genuine uncertainty as to the effectiveness of a treatment.

At the end of the trial, researchers look to see what the differences in outcome are between the different groups in the trial – for example, what was the difference in weight loss between the groups who received different interventions. Because the groups were otherwise equal, we can say that any difference in outcome (for example weight loss) is likely to be attributable to the intervention.

What is a 'null' hypothesis?

A null hypothesis is usually stated when an RCT is designed. The null hypothesis states that there is no difference between the two groups. The aim of the

RCT is to determine whether the null hypothesis can be confirmed or rejected. If the results show that there is a difference between the control group and the intervention group, then the null hypothesis can be rejected.

A flow diagram of the process of conducting an RCT for weight loss programme is presented below:

> Poster is sited in a weight loss clinic for those interested in entering a trial to compare weight loss treatments.
> ↓
> People who respond to the advertisement and fit the inclusion criteria become the sample. This population is randomly allocated into two groups:
> ↓
> 1 Group one receives the new weight loss intervention strategy.
> 2 Group two receive standard clinic treatment.
> ↓
> The rate of weight loss is compared between the two groups. Any differences in outcomes is attributed to the different treatments given that the groups were randomised.

Example: Diggle and Deeks (2006) conducted an RCT to explore whether needle size used in the vaccination of infants had any effect on the extent of the local reaction experienced after vaccination. They divided their sample of infants into two random groups – one group was vaccinated using one needle size and the other group using a different needle size and the reaction experienced by the infants was observed. Using this process, Diggle and Deeks found that using the longer needle significantly reduced local reaction.

Quasi experiments

Quasi experiments have some of the features of an RCT but not all of them. They are not a true experiment.

 Quasi experiments are most useful when . . . you need to find out if something is effective, but are not able to undertake a randomised controlled trial.

When do you use a quasi experiment?

A quasi experiment might be the best approach available, when it is not possible to undertake an RCT. This may be because it is not possible to randomise participants or because it is not possible to withhold treatment from one group of participants. For example, if you were exploring infant nutrition, it would not be acceptable or ethical to ask one group of mothers to abstain from breast-feeding their babies in order to make a comparison with another group of mothers who were asked to breast feed.

Example: imagine you want to find out whether a new style of parenting class is effective. Because of the nature of child care, it is not possible to undertake an RCT. Instead you implement the new style of class with one group of parents who have enrolled on a parenting class and compare the results with another group in another area who have not completed this class . . . You can see that the two groups in the experiment are not equal – the parents in one class might come from different sociological groups than those in another and whilst you might allow for this by selecting similar areas to take part in the study, you will not achieve equal groups as you would in an RCT. Therefore if the outcomes for the parents who experienced the new style of parenting class were different from the outcomes of those who did not, you cannot tell if these outcomes would be different due to other factors.

Therefore in a quasi experiment, it is not possible to say with as much certainty that the outcome was due to the intervention administered. Whilst non-randomised experiments will provide you with evidence, this is generally thought to be **second best evidence** if you are looking to determine the evidence of effectiveness.

Cohort studies and case control studies

Cohort studies and case control studies are studies that try to link up the causes of diseases and/or interventions and/or social situations. Cohort studies and case control studies were first used to observe the effects of an exposure (say smoking) on the health of those observed.

Cohort and case control studies are most useful when . . . you need information about the likely causes of disease and other problems. For example, you wonder whether those using illicit drugs are more likely to present in the accident and emergency department on a Saturday evening than on other days.

What is a cohort study?

Cohort studies are observational studies. These studies attempt to discover the causes of disease or problem when it is not possible to carry out an RCT.

A cohort study is the study of a group of people who have all been exposed to a particular event or lifestyle (for example let's say that they all smoke).

- They have been used most often to find the causes or impact of disease.
- They are then followed up in order to observe the effect of the exposure to – for example – smoking nicotine on the health and social wellbeing of those observed.

Example: a cohort study published in 2009 was able to identify that women who drink even modest amounts of alcohol are more at risk of developing breast cancer than their non-drinking counterparts. Women attending a clinic for breast cancer screening were followed up and the drinking habits of those who went on to develop breast cancer were compared to those who did not develop the disease. This cohort study demonstrated that there was a strong association between alcohol consumption and development of breast cancer.

A flow diagram of the process of conducting a cohort study is presented below:

Cohort of people who all experienced the same exposure/experience.

↓

This cohort are followed up to observe the effect of this exposure.

They may be compared to the control group who did not experience this exposure, but because the groups were not formed by random allocation, any observed differences between the two groups at the end of the study period is not as easily attributable to the exposure as if the study had been an RCT.

What is a case control study?

 A case control study is one in which patient/clients with a particular condition are studied and compared with others who do not have that condition in order to try to establish whether a particular exposure has caused led to a condition.

Example: 'does poor housing lead to asthma?'

- A case control study works the other way round to a cohort study. Cases that have a condition are studied and compared to cases that do not. You could for example explore the alcohol consumption of those who have developed breast cancer and compare this against those who do not have the disease.
- It is useful where it may be unethical to use RCTs.

Example: In 1954, Doll and Hill carried out a case control study examining lung cancer. In their study, patient/clients were traced back to see what could have caused the disease. They designed a questionnaire which was given to patient/clients with suspected lung, liver or bowel cancer. Those administering the questionnaire were not aware which of the diseases was suspected in which patient/clients. It became clear from the questionnaires that those who were later confirmed to have lung cancer were also confirmed smokers. Those who did not have lung cancer did not smoke. Clearly it would not have been ethical to have undertaken an RCT to explore the causes of lung cancer as it would not have been possible to randomise a group of non-smokers and ask one group to start smoking!

A flow diagram of the process of conducting a case control study is presented below:

Individuals with a specific condition or situation are identified.
↓
The circumstances that led up to the development/progress of this condition are then explored.

Questionnaire/surveys/cross-sectional studies

Questionnaire/surveys are studies in which a sample is taken at *any one point in time* (cross-section of a population) from *a defined group of people* and observed/assessed.

Data can be either quantitative (asking specific questions) or qualitative (asking open questions).

Questionnaire/surveys are most useful when . . . you are looking for evidence about frequency of a particular activity, or information about a large group of people. Remember that questionnaire/survey studies have many limitations as outlined below and the results of these should be viewed with caution.

Boynton and Greenhalgh (2004) comment on the ease with which questionnaires are distributed without ensuring that the questionnaire will provide useful data. They discuss the frequent use of poorly designed questionnaires that lack rigour and hence lead to the collection of poor quality data and subsequently to misleading conclusions.

For a questionnaire to be useful, researchers must know in advance what questions they need to ask. If very little is known about a particular area, further exploratory work may need to be done prior to the development of the questionnaire. A questionnaire will only collect useful data if the questions have been well tested and piloted. This is to ensure that the questions mean the same thing to those who respond as they do to those who designed them. This will also include how the questions are presented. Even with the best designed questionnaire, unless it is distributed to a representative sample of the population, the quality of the results will be reduced. It is very difficult to achieve a random sample in a questionnaire survey which is distributed face to face as only those in attendance on that day have the possibility to respond to a questionnaire. A postal questionnaire can be distributed to a **random sample** of the population but it is highly unlikely that everyone will respond. This affects the quality of the data as it is not known how the responses from those who did not respond would have differed from those who did. It is equally very difficult to achieve a random sample in a postal questionnaire as the response rates tend to be low.

If it is possible to distribute a questionnaire face to face, you may achieve a higher response rate, but you will not achieve a random sample, as you are only selecting participants from those patient/clients attending on a particular day.

Example: if you distributed the questionnaire in a shopping centre on a Saturday, you would reach a different population than if the questionnaire was distributed on a weekday. Similarly, you would be likely to get a different group of people depending on the time at which the questionnaire was distributed.

Example: A questionnaire to explore the incidence of illicit drug use at one point in time.

- The purpose of a **cross-sectional study** is to provide a snapshot illustration of the attributes of a given population in the sample.
- The evidence they contain is therefore likely to be less strong than other forms of evidence.
- Cross-sectional studies are not strong evidence for establishing the effectiveness of interventions but are useful for measuring specific actions, attitudes and behaviours of a given group of people.
- **Questionnaire/surveys** are printed lists of questions used to find out information from people.
- They can be used as a means of data collection in RCTs, cohort and case control studies and other studies.
- They are often used to find out specific information from people at one point in time only.
- The nature of the questions asked can provide descriptive data, for example: *How many university students use illicit drugs on campus?*
- Alternatively, some further analysis can be attempted, for example: *Do all those who report using Class A drugs also report early illicit drug use?*

How useful is data collected from a questionnaire/survey?

It is very difficult to design and implement a good questionnaire/survey study. The development of a questionnaire is difficult and the information obtained is highly dependent on the quality of the questionnaire developed. Data collected from a questionnaire can be unreliable for the following reasons:

- A long questionnaire might be discarded before completion.
- Complicated or badly worded questions may be misunderstood by the respondent.
- Postal questionnaires have the additional disadvantage that there is likely to be a low response rate.
- It is often not possible to get access to fully representative sample for the distribution of a questionnaire.
- The completed questionnaires will contain information from a selection of, but not a random sample, of participants and will therefore give an incomplete picture of the target population.
- Any apparent associations arising from the analysis of questionnaire data should be interpreted with caution. For example, if it was identified that those who used illicit drugs also experienced high anxiety levels, it would be tempting to conclude that use of illicit drugs increases student anxiety. However perhaps the reverse is true and that those with high levels of anxiety resort to illicit drug use.
- If large sections of the target population do not respond, the overall quality of data that is collected will be poor.

Sampling in quantitative research

The sample will be taken from the wider population to whom the research project relates.

Example: a sample of university students could be taken from the university population as a whole.

Sample size in quantitative research tends to be large. This is because researchers are concerned with validity; that is, whether the findings of a study are valid or reflect reality.

Example: you are likely to have greater confidence in a study comparing two treatment options in which many thousands of people had participated than a study conducted on just twenty participants.

Think of a questionnaire or survey you have completed. Consider how appropriate was the sample size involved in the research?

If the condition under investigation is unusual, sample sizes will inevitably be smaller. However paradoxically, you need to get big numbers in a study to be able to find out about the incidence rate.

Random sampling is often used in quantitative research. Random sampling is defined as meaning that all those in the sample have an **equal chance of being selected** in the sample. This ensures that the sample is not biased.

Example: a random sample of university students could be drawn from the university admission lists rather than from the attendance at lectures, given that all students will be on the admission list, but not all will attend lectures. Any sample drawn from those who attend lectures will be biased rather than random. It is important to note that obtaining an unbiased sample in any research study is very difficult. A questionnaire might be sent to a random sample of the population, but unless there is a 100% **response rate**, the responses obtained will be biased.

Some studies use **random allocation** within a non-random sample, rather than random sampling overall.

Example: in an RCT the selected group (**convenience sample**) may be patient/clients attending a particular clinic, who will then be randomised into different intervention groups.

Data analysis in quantitative research

There are two types of statistics: descriptive and inferential.

Descriptive statistics describe the data given in the paper. These statistics should clearly describe the main results.

Example: how many people answered 'yes' to a particular question, or what the most common response to a question was.
The results will typically be given using the

Mean: this is the average when all the results are added up and divided by the number of participants. **Example:** if results from 5 participants were 25, 35, 20, 20 40 then the average score would be the total of this (140) divided by the number of participants (5) (= an average score of 28).

Median: the middle value if the results are ranked from lowest to highest.

Example: in 11 results as follows 1, 1, 2, 3, 3, **4**, 5, 6, 6, 7, 7 the number 4 is in the middle.

Mode: this is the number that occurs most often so in 1,1, 2, 3, 3, 3, 6, 7, 8, 8, then 3 is the mode as it occurs three times.

Percentages are also used. This indicates how many out of 100 such as 65%.

Inferential statistics generalise to the wider population. In other words, to determine the extent to which the results obtained from the sample in the research have any relevance to the **wider population** as a whole.

- Inferential statistics do more than describe a sample, they infer from it to the wider population.
- The bigger the sample, the surer you can be that the sample prevalence is close to the population prevalence.

Example: at the time of a general election, opinion polls are used to predict the overall result of the election. These polls are based on a small sample of voters but are used with good accuracy to predict the overall result.

Confidence intervals

The confidence we can have that the sample is an accurate indication of the true population prevalence is reflected in **confidence intervals**.

- The smaller the interval or range, the more confident you can be that the results in the study reflect the results you would find in the larger population.
- Using a formula, the confidence intervals, upper and lower are calculated. A **95% confidence interval** means that we can be 95% sure that the true population prevalence lies between the lower and upper confidence interval.

Probability value (p value)

Statistics are often described as a **p value** or probability value. The p value expresses the probability of the difference shown between the groups in an experiment being due to chance. It is important to determine the likelihood that the findings are down to chance in any research.

The lower the p value the less likely it is that the occurrence is due to chance. If a p value is less than 0.05 (1:20) we say the occurrence is unlikely to be due to chance. If the p value is much less that 0.05 (1:20) for example p = 0.005 (1:200) then the occurrence is even more unlikely to be due to chance.

Example: you are undertaking an RCT comparing different ways to help people stop smoking. Normally in an RCT, you would give an intervention to one group and not to the other and then examine the differences in outcomes between the groups.

If however, both groups were treated with the standard treatment you would likely see a variety of outcomes in each group due to natural differences between the groups. Then, you administer an intervention to one of the groups and observe the different outcomes of the two groups. The p value can then be calculated to determine whether the differences in outcomes observed is due to chance or not.

To calculate the p value we use the **null hypothesis**. This is a phrase that is used when you state (in order to test it) that there is no relationship between the different elements (or **variables**) under study. This can be calculated using a statistical test, such as the Chi squared test. A p value of 0.05, for example, means there is a (1:20) chance of seeing these results if the null hypothesis were true. So, this means that there is a relationship between the variables. It is important to remember that this does not indicate a causal relationship, i.e. that one variable caused the other, but just that the two occur together.

Qualitative studies

The principle of all qualitative approaches is to explore the meaning of and **develop in-depth understanding** of the research topic as experienced by the participants of the research.

Qualitative research is most useful when . . . you are looking for in-depth answers to questions that cannot be answered numerically. When you are asking why? or how? or what? You are likely to be looking at qualitative research to find answers to your question.

Think of an area of your own practice where you could explore a qualitative question relating to the experience of, or understanding of, an issue.

Qualitative studies typically **do not seek to quantify or measure** the items under exploration using numbers – an approach which lies traditionally in the quantitative domain, in which the measurements taken by the researchers are repeatable and re-testable.

The aim of most qualitative data analysis is:

- To study the interview scripts or other data obtained for the study and to **develop an understanding** of this data.
- The data is **coded** and **themes** are then generated from the data set.
- The generation of themes, although rigorous, is **interpretative and subjective**, depending on the insight of the researcher.

The search for evidence of rigour in qualitative research is difficult due to the interpretative and exploratory nature of qualitative studies. It can therefore be difficult for those who critique a qualitative study to determine the strengths and limitations of the study.

The most commonly used **data collection methods** in qualitative research are:

- In-depth interviews
- Focus groups
- Questionnaires using open ended questions.

Large numbers of participants are rarely used (and are not necessarily appropriate) in qualitative research.

The richness of qualitative data arises from **the dialogue between the researcher and the researched** and the insights obtained through this process are only possible because of the **interaction** between the two. **Example**, the interviewer may probe the interviewee about his or her responses to a question and phrases the next question as a direct response to the reply received. **Subjectivity is required** for the researcher to get an insight into the topic of investigation and objectivity is not strived for.

Qualitative data analysis is **open to interpretation**. Because the researcher is involved in, and indeed shapes, both the data collection and analysis process, it is not possible for the researcher to remain detached from the data which is collected. The concept of **reflexivity** refers to the acknowledgement by the qualitative researcher that this process of enquiry is necessarily open to interpretation and that **detachment** from the focus of the research is **neither desirable nor possible**.

What are the characteristics of qualitative research?

- **Depth** rather than breadth is the focus of qualitative research.
- Researchers seek to understand the *whole* of an experience and insight of the situation.

- The data collected is not numerical but is collected, often through interview, using the words and descriptions given by participants.
- There is no use of statistics in qualitative research; the results are descriptive and interpretative.
- Sample sizes tend to be **small**. A small sample is required because in-depth understanding (rather than statistical analysis) is sought from information-rich participants who take part. For this reason, a small sample size should be regarded as appropriate in qualitative research. This is in contrast to quantitative research in which the nearer the sample size is to the true population, the more representative the results will be. Russell and Gregory (2003) argue that different qualitative approaches require different sample sizes and advise that phenomenological studies tend to have smaller samples than grounded theory studies or ethnographic studies. When you are reviewing a study it is important to consider the account given by the researchers.
- They do not set out looking for specific ideas, hoping to confirm pre-existing beliefs. Instead, they code the data according to ideas arising from within it. This process is often referred to as **inductive**.
- Researchers do not generally strive to achieve objectivity because this would strip away the context from the topic of research.
- The researcher cannot achieve complete objectivity because he or she is the data collection tool (for example, the interviewer) and interprets the data that is collected. This is acknowledged in the research process and steps are taken to maintain objectivity as far as possible.
- This research is sometimes referred to as naturalistic research.
- The participants used in a qualitative study, tend not to be selected at random, instead participants are selected if they have had exposure to or experience of the phenomenon of interest in the particular study. This type of sampling is referred to as **purposive sampling** and this leads to the selection of information rich cases who can contribute to the answering of the research question. Other approaches to sampling in qualitative research are **theoretical** – where the sample is determined according to the needs of the study and snowball sampling – where the sample is developed as new potential participants are identified as the study progresses. For example, the contacts of participants already involved in the research may be invited to enter the study, if they have the relevant experience.
- Qualitative data is analysed by coding the data and building themes.

Example of qualitative research questions

- What it is like for a patient/client who has had a stroke?
- What is it like to be forced to leave one's own home due to repossession?
- How do patient/clients with newly diagnosed diabetes cope with their condition?
- Why do independent nurse prescribers prescribe less than general practitioners?

Are there different approaches to qualitative research?

Yes. There are a wide variety of approaches to qualitative research. You are likely to encounter many different approaches to qualitative research when you read the literature. Some are just described in the literature as 'qualitative studies' whilst others are named according to the particular qualitative approach that is followed. These are outlined below. It is useful to recognise these different approaches and to understand why one approach was selected for a specific research question.

Grounded theory is a way of finding out about what happens in a social setting and then making wider generalisations about the way things happen. It is a 'bottom up' approach in which data is collected and analysed and then used to make explanations about the way things happen in social life.

Example: why do people start smoking – data is collected from those who smoke and then used to make wider generalisations to the population as a whole.

Phenomenology is the study of the 'lived experience' or what it is actually like to live with a particular condition or experience. These studies often use in depth interviews as the means of data collection as they allow the participant the opportunity to explore and describe their experience within an interview setting.

Example: what is it like for a child to visit a parent in prison?

Ethnography is the study of human culture. An ethnographic study focusses on a community (i.e. a specific group of people) in order to gain insight about how its members behave. Observation or participant observation and/or in-depth interviews may be undertaken to achieve this. As it seeks to observe phenomena as it occurs in real time a true ethnographic study is a time consuming process.

Example: what is life like living rough on the streets?

Action research is the process by which practitioners or researchers work together to address issues that arise in everyday practice in order to develop a systematic approach to change implementation and the evaluation of change. Action research is a cyclical method of planning, implementing and evaluating change and development in the working environment. For example, Elliott (2003) explored the use of portfolios in an action research project designed to look at the development of continuing professional development within a social care setting. Changes in the use of the portfolio as a tool for continuing professional development were introduced and evaluated in the action research project.

Action research is most useful when . . . you need to generate improvements in organisations that are not in the form of research findings, but are generated as solutions from within.

- It is often designed and conducted by practitioners who analyse the data to improve their own practice.
- It can be done by individuals or by teams of colleagues in the workplace.
- Other means of data collection include focus groups and direct observation.

 After reading this section, try and summarise your learning on literature reviews, quantitative and qualitative research methodologies. If you are unclear, read the section again or discuss it with a colleague/fellow student.

Which type of research is best?

There has been much debate in the research literature about the merits of different approaches to research (i.e. quantitative or qualitative) with some researchers claiming that one is better than another. In this book we argue that these debates are not important.

 What is important is that the most **appropriate research methodology** is used to address the **research question**.

The varied research methods are outlined below in order to illustrate that it is no good using qualitative methods to address a question where quantitative methods are more appropriate or vice versa. It is important that you can access this information to address the decisions you make in practice.

There are many similarities between both approaches to research. Both commence with a research question and select the appropriate methodology to answer this question. In all research papers, the methods used to undertake the research should be clearly explained and the results clearly presented. This is known as the **research process**.

I have read about the term 'hierarchy of evidence'. What does it mean?

There is general agreement that a hierarchy of evidence exists and that some forms of research evidence are stronger than others in addressing different types of questions.

There is a traditional hierarchy of evidence which puts systematic reviews and randomised controlled trials at the top and qualitative studies at the bottom as shown below.

Example hierarchy of evidence for determining effective treatment

1. Systematic reviews and meta-analyses	Highest
2. Randomised controlled trials	
3. Cohort studies, case controlled studies	
4. Surveys	
5. Case reports	
6. Qualitative studies	
7. Expert opinion	
8. Anecdotal opinion	Lowest

(Sackett *et al.* 1996)

Hierarchies such as this can be misleading because they are only relevant if you are looking for evidence to determine whether a treatment or intervention is effective or not.

In many areas of health and social care, the traditional hierarchy is not appropriate for exploring complex questions. You are not only interested in finding out whether something is effective or not; there are many other questions you need to address. We have emphasised throughout this book that it is important that you work out what type of information you need and you should seek this information in the first instance. In a previous publication, Aveyard (2007) refers to making up **your own 'hierarchy of evidence'** that you need to address your own particular research question. This is because the traditional hierarchy of evidence only applies when you are looking for evidence of effectiveness. It is derived from a medical model that does not apply when the area to be researched is not concerned with effectiveness of interventions.

Some examples of selecting the right research approach in order to answer the question:

Example 1: Evidence about effectiveness. If you need to find out about the effectiveness of one dressing over another (or of anything else) you would need to look for RCTs which have compared the two dressings (or whatever it is you are looking for). This is because this will enable you to determine whether one dressing was more effective than another. Therefore, RCTs would be top of your hierarchy in this instance for the evidence you are looking for. If available a systematic review of RCTs would be even better.

Example 2: Evidence about incidence of disease or situations. If you need to find out whether those people taking a particular drug are more at risk of a particular condition (let's take for example thalidomide which was prescribed in the 1960s to pregnant women as an anti-sickness medication), you would need to look for case controlled trials or cohort studies which has explored the effects of a particular exposure on the population in question. Therefore cohort studies or case control studies would be at the top of the hierarchy in this instance for the evidence you are looking for.

Example 3: Evidence about vulnerable families. If you want to find out how health and social care professionals undertake the assessment of vulnerable families, you would need to find evidence of what happens in practice by descriptions of care undertaken, or better still of observations of the care delivered. Therefore qualitative studies of observation of or accounts of care delivery would be at the top of your hierarchy of evidence in this instance.

Example 4: Evidence about social life. If you want to find out what it is like to enter the UK as a migrant worker, you would need to find evidence of the experience of those workers. Therefore, qualitative studies, probably using a phenomenological account would be at the top of your hierarchy of evidence in this instance.

Example 5: Evidence about student life. If you wanted to find out how many students use illicit drugs whilst at university, you would need to find questionnaires/surveys which have explored this aspect of student life. Whilst the data collected from questionnaires can be unreliable, in this instance, there is really no other way to get at this data. Therefore, this data would be at the top of your hierarchy of evidence in this instance.

From these examples you can see that when you have established what it is you need to find out, you can then determine the type of evidence you are looking for which will enable you to find out what you need to know.

What about using secondary sources?

Secondary sources often comment on the original or primary sources in order to summarise large or hard to access information.

A secondary source is a source that is a step removed from the ideas you are referring to.

Example: a report in the *British Medical Journal* (BMJ) might refer to a systematic review published by the Cochrane Collaboration. The BMJ report would be the secondary source and the Cochrane Collaboration report the primary source.

- You are advised to access the primary source wherever possible and the use of secondary sources should be avoided wherever possible.
- If you rely on a secondary report and you do not access the original report, there is potential for error in the way in which the initial source was reported and interpreted.
- Therefore where you need to quote an author directly, you are always advised to access this original paper rather than to refer to a report of it, unless it is not possible to get hold of the primary source, for example if it is out of print or an unpublished doctoral thesis.

Example: let's say that the author of a paper you are reading (author 1) cites the work of another author (author 2) who has done work in the area. If you refer to the work of author 2 without accessing the original work this is a secondary source and should be avoided. This is because unless you read the original work by author 2 directly, you are relying on another author's interpretation of this work. This means that you cannot comment on the way it is represented by author 1, the full context or upon the strengths and limitations of the original work.

Professional and clinical guidance

In addition to empirical research, there is a range of guidelines and policies that are available. Ideally, these guidelines and policies are developed from the best available evidence. They should be written in a user friendly way so that you can apply the evidence easily in your professional setting. There is a wide range of local, national and international guidance available for health and social care professionals. There are also clinical and professional guidelines specific to individual professions and sometimes clinical disorders. It is worth accessing societies, colleges and organisations specific to your profession.

This information might be used

- To give you a broad background/overview of your topic.
- To see what current opinion/debate is surrounding the topic.
- To add context to your introduction and discussion chapters if you are writing up your review of the literature, especially when the results of empirical studies conflict.

A range of guides is available at: http://www.library.nhs.uk/Default.aspx

They are categorised into the following sections which are discussed in detail below:

- **Clinical knowledge summaries**
- **National library of guidelines**
- **Map of medicine health guides**

Clinical knowledge summaries (CKS) incorporating Prodigy. This collection is defined as a reliable source of evidence based information and practical 'know how' about the common conditions managed in primary care. Its aim is to provide quick answers to real-life questions that arise, linking to detailed answers that clearly outline the evidence on which they are based.

The national library of guidelines is a collection of guidelines for the NHS. It is based on the guidelines produced by the National Institute for Health and Clinical Excellence (NICE) http://www.nice.org.uk/ and other national agencies. NICE describes itself as an independent organisation responsible for providing national guidance on promoting good health and preventing and treating ill health. There have, however, been some criticisms of its approach particularly as it may be seen to be used as a way of rationing care.

They mainly focus on guidelines produced in the UK, where available, if not then guidelines from other countries are used. They have strict inclusion criteria.

NICE issues guidelines of very high quality.

- They are based on a systematic review of the evidence and have extensive consultation not only with clinicians but also with patients and, where relevant, industry.
- Professional associations do not have the resources to carry out this type of consultation but they can follow the principles set out in the **AGREE**

protocol available at http://www.agreecollaboration.org/ which helps guideline writers minimise bias, meet the needs of all stakeholders and maximise clarity.

Map of medicine health guides is a web-based visual representation of evidence-based patient care journeys covering 28 medical specialties and over 350 pathways. Available at http://healthguides.mapofmedicine.com/choices/map/index.html.

Non-research based evidence

As we have stated before, there will not always be evidence available for the area you seek. In this case, you may use weaker evidence (such as expert opinion, discussion papers and so on) to address the question you seek to answer. In this case, it is especially important that you assess the quality of the evidence that you have as we will discuss in Chapter 6.

Example: a discussion article written by a leading expert in a particular area might be considered to carry more weight than a similar article written by a student.

In summary

There is a wide range of research evidence that you are likely to encounter when you seek evidence to answer questions that arise in your practice. It is important that you can recognise different types of research and understand when and why different approaches are used.

We will discuss how you search for and make sense of what you come across in the next two chapters. It is important that you are aware that different types of research evidence will assist you in addressing different types of questions that arise in practice.

Key points

1 You are likely to encounter a wide range of research and other information that is relevant to your clinical question.

2 Traditional hierarchies of evidence only apply if you are looking for evidence of effectiveness.
3 It is important to identify the types of research and other information that you need to address your question.
4 You may come across a wide range of evidence – what is important is that you can recognise what you read and use it appropriately.

5

How do I find the evidence to support my practice and learning?

How do I focus the topic area and ask the right question? • Focussing and structuring your question using PICOT • How do I search for literature? • Developing a comprehensive approach to searching for literature • Potential problems with haphazard/casual approaches to finding literature • Steps in the search process • 1. State the focus of your literature search • 2. Identify your key terms • 3. Define your inclusion and exclusion criteria • 4. Undertaking a comprehensive search • 5. Recording your searching strategy • 6. Manage and store your literature effectively • In summary • Key points

In this chapter we will consider

- What evidence to look for – identifying your focus/keywords/search terms
- How to use the internet, databases and library
- How to search and how to increase, refine or reduce the results of a search
- How to use more advanced searching – limits and tips
- Using experts, specialists and colleagues
- What to include and what to reject.

How do I focus the topic area and ask the right question?

You may have a broad idea of the topic, relating to a decision you have made or need to make, but have yet to identify what exactly you need to focus on in order to focus your question. You may have a more specific interest in mind which has arisen from your academic studies or assignment you need to write. We have already emphasised that the evidence you search for will depend on the question you need to answer. Therefore you need to refine and focus the question you need to answer before you start searching for evidence.

Remember: different questions require different evidence!

Your ideas to explore the evidence base for a clinical issue or problem could come from a variety of sources as previously discussed and this will depend on the nature of the question you want to address. In Chapter 2 we discussed the information revolution and how as professionals we are inundated with information about our practice. This is why it is important to have a narrow focus for the question you want to ask.

If you undertake searches on large topics such as diabetes, or a clinical problem such as depression, immobility or even an intervention such as wound dressings you will get too large a number of results (hits) from your search.

 It is important to be really clear about **what you want to find out** before you start looking in order to be more efficient with your time.

Consider what area of practice you are exploring. Your enquiry may relate to: assessment, screening, diagnosis, prognosis, prevention, interventions, management, outcomes, cost-benefits, patient/client/service user or staff or student experience, and so on.

There are many approaches you can take when you are **starting to define the question** you want to ask. These include:

- Thinking through/reflecting on your practice to isolate what really concerns you
- Talking to experts
- Brainstorming ideas with colleagues
- Using a spider diagram or mind map
- Carrying out a quick initial database search
- Using a search engine to see broadly what terms/subjects come up
- Google Scholar can be a good place to start (available as a drop down menu on the 'more' tab on the front page of Google).

When you focus on the question you need to answer, this means that you ask a specific question rather than seeking information about the entire topic. You have probably found this already when undertaking search engine searches (such as GOOGLE). If you ask for information on a particular country or event, you may get thousands of hits. When you refine this to something more specific you probably come nearer to finding what you are looking for. It is the same within health and social care. If you are searching for information on a topic, you need to know exactly what you are trying to find out.

Example: if you were searching for information on needle size in the administration of vaccines, you would need to search for this specifically, rather than the rather large topic of vaccinations. Consider the aspect of your topic that you really need to explore and define the question you need to ask.

Example: if you were looking for evidence about the outcomes for children at risk who were moved out of the family home, then you would need to look specifically at these children rather than children at risk who were not removed from the home.

Example: if you are wondering why your patient/client's leg ulcer is not responding to the treatment you are giving. You have heard that using manuka honey might be effective in the healing process. You want to explore this. You frame the question you need to answer as something like this – '*how effective is manuka honey in healing leg ulcers?*'

Framed like this, you know that you need to seek information only that is related to manuka honey and its healing properties and will not get sidelined by other more general information you encounter if it is not related to the healing properties of manuka honey.

Focussing and structuring your question using PICOT

Consider using the acronym **PICOT** when you are identifying the question you want to address. Do note that the sections of PICOT have different meanings depending on whether you are looking for quantitative or qualitative research. Fineout-Overholt and Johnson (2005) suggest the two following stages of defining a question, depending on the type of research we are looking for:

Standard PICOT	**Qualitative PICOT**
Population	Population
Intervention	Issue

Comparison   Context
Outcome   Outcome
Time   Time

Population: We need to consider who are the people we are interested in investigating with similar characteristics such as gender, age, condition, problem, location, role, e.g. older people in residential care, those who are homeless, mothers under 45, patient/clients who have had knee replacements, patient/clients who have accessed paramedic services for chest pain, staff who work out of hours, students who access study advice.

Intervention/issue (quantitative/qualitative): These can be diagnostic, therapeutic, preventative, exposure, managerial, experiences, perceptions, costs and so on.

Comparisons/context (quantitative/qualitative): This can be against another intervention or no intervention, comparisons can be made against national or professional standards or guidelines. The context of the study can be where the study takes place.

Outcome: Faster, cheaper, reasons why, reduction or increase in, for example: symptoms, benefits, events, episodes, prognosis, mortality, accuracy.

Time: This may or may not be relevant, for example: 3 days postoperative or 5 hours post-intervention, within 24 hours of accessing the service.

Example of PICOT question (quantitative): Does education about smoking *(intervention)* **reduce smoking** *(outcome)* **in young people** *(population)* **in state education** *(context and comparison if there is a control group of those who did not receive education)* **before the age of 16** *(time)*?

Example of PICOT question (qualitative): Why *(outcome)* **do young people** *(population)* **in state education** *(context)* **start smoking** *(issue)* **before the age of 16** *(time)*?

 Activity: Try writing a research question using the PICOT process on something you want to explore in your practice.

Once you have identified what you are looking to find out, you need to consider what evidence will enable you to answer the question. Whilst appreciating which research approaches are most likely to be relevant to answering your research question, you are advised to remain open-minded at this stage about the inclusion of all types of information if they are relevant to your research question otherwise you risk losing important data (Lloyd-Jones 2004).

Remember . . .

You need to determine what evidence you need to answer your question. A single source of evidence that has not been 'judged' or appraised for its quality is generally not enough.

We will consider this aspect further as we go through this book.

How do I search for literature?

Once you have established the question you want to answer (**research question**) you need to develop an effective approach to your search (**search strategy**) that will enable you to identify and locate the widest range and most relevant publications within your time and financial limitations.

The main approach to literature searching is likely to be using academic **electronic databases** held in your local library. You should become familiar with your local library and its facilities. However you will also use other searching strategies which we will discuss.

Developing a comprehensive approach to searching for literature (developing a search strategy or methodology)

This is a key area – if you are comprehensive or systematic in your approach to searching for literature, you are likely to get access to a comprehensive range of literature.

If you do not adopt a systematic approach, you are likely to get access to a random selection of literature. A comprehensive or systematic approach to searching includes both where you search (databases and other sources) and what you search for (key terms).

- **Potential problems with Google?** Internet search engines such as Google are **not** specific enough to effectively search although they may give you some ideas of terms language used. This is why you need to access a **subject specific search engine or database**.

- A literature search that is approached systematically is very different from one that is approached in a haphazard manner!
- A thorough and comprehensive search strategy will help to ensure that you identify all the key literature/texts and research on your topic.
- If you are using the information to share with others or in your writing then documenting your stated strategy will ensure that those who access your evidence know what you looked for, what was included, excluded and where you searched.

 Think about how you might have accessed literature in the past for your learning and for your practice and consider the pros and cons of these approaches.

You may have found literature in your workplace, from a search engine or website or obtained it from colleagues. Or you might have carried out a quick search and used the first thing you found.

Potential problems with haphazard/casual approaches to finding literature

- It could be out of date.
- It could be biased.
- You may miss out on finding key literature.
- It may not be the best available evidence for the question you have.
- Contradictory literature may be out there.
- It may present only one part of the whole picture.
- Harder-to-find literature may be really useful in answering your question.
- Your conclusions are likely to be inaccurate.

Steps in the search process

1 State the focus of the literature that you will seek – the research question.
2 Identify your key terms and inclusion and exclusion criteria.
3 Define inclusion and exclusion criteria.
4 Undertake a comprehensive search using your key terms and inclusion and exclusion criteria.

5 Record your search strategy.
6 Manage and store your literature effectively.

1. State the focus of your literature search

If you articulate your focus at the beginning of the searching process, this will help to keep you on track. It is important to ensure that you only find that information which is relevant to the research question and it is very easy to get sidetracked so it is suggested you use PICOT as described above to form a clear question.

2. Identify your key terms

Once you have articulated the focus of your literature search, you need to identify some key terms for which you can search for literature. You need to think laterally when you do this – try and think of the different ways in which your topic could be referred to and identify the keywords that you think are likely to represent your topic. This is one time when using Google can help you to do this – as you will see the different ways that your topic is discussed and the phrases that are used. You can also use the thesaurus component of a database search engine. You can also refer to other published literature in the area to find out how the authors of other papers have searched using keywords. You will find that your search for evidence is not a one-off process but an evolving process that you return to and refine as your ideas develop.

- You should be as creative as possible as the topic or question might be categorised in different ways by different researchers.
- Think of all the words that may mean the same thing (use a thesaurus if you can, they are often accessible on the database itself).
- Consider different spellings of the same word (US and UK) and/or if the endings may vary i.e. children/child/children's (see below).
- You also need to consider whether there are different meanings in different countries to the keywords that you identify, especially given that databases have different biases. For example, CINAHL has a strong North American bias, the BNI has a British focus.
- Don't limit your keywords to terms that are conventional if you think literature might be indexed using different headings.
- You will find that you identify new possible search terms as your searching progresses.

Example: Consider the way in which the term 'learning difficulties/disabilities' is used. Some people have strong feelings about which term is used. However, if you are searching for literature in this area, be careful to use every term that might have been used to index the literature or you risk omitting vital literature from your search.

3. Define your inclusion and exclusion criteria

 Inclusion and exclusion criteria enable you to identify the literature that addresses the research question and to reject that which does not.

Once you have identified your key terms, you need to identify inclusion and exclusion criteria that will assist you in selecting appropriate literature for your topic. Whilst inclusion and exclusion criteria are generally used by those undertaking a search as part of a larger more formal literature review, the principles of including and excluding relevant/irrelevant literature apply to every literature search.

- The criteria you develop will be guided by the wording of your research question and your focus.
- Unless your question clearly indicates otherwise, you are likely to be looking for primary research or literature reviews in the first instance.
- You should be able to justify why you have set the inclusion and exclusion criteria, which should be determined by the needs of the question you need to answer rather than your own convenience. For example, it would not be appropriate to include only studies which are accessed electronically if a hard paper copy of an article you require is available in the local library.

Example **of inclusion criteria:**

- Primary research directly related to the topic
- English language only
- Published literature only
- 1995 onwards
- In a particular setting or a particular population

Example **of exclusion criteria:**

- Primary research not directly related to the topic area
- Non-English language
- Unpublished research

- Pre-1995
- Not in a particular setting or with a particular population

Should I limit my search for practical reasons?

In an ideal world, you would be able to search and locate all the information that is relevant to your question. However, some of your criteria will be set for practical reasons, such as time and resources; for example, limiting your search to recent literature and to omit unpublished literature from your search. Neither of these restrictions are ideal and you might lose relevant literature – for example, there might be a piece of work which is highly relevant to your review but which was published before the date limitations you set. If you set time restrictions to your search for literature you would miss this key document, although it might be referred to in other papers.

Should I limit my search to published literature only?

Again, in an ideal world, you would seek to access all available literature on your topic. There is also concern about reviewing only literature that has been published. This is because of the risk of publication bias; that is journals tend to publish research that shows the positive effect of an intervention rather than a negative effect or no effect (Easterbrook *et al.* 1991). There might be a lot of 'hidden' evidence about your topic that remains unpublished (called 'grey literature') because the results showed no effect. Non-academic journals might also be referred to as grey literature and other information such as policies also fall into this category.

4. Undertaking a comprehensive search

Once you have identified your question, keywords and inclusion and exclusion criteria, you are ready to begin searching for literature/evidence.
   There are five main ways of searching for literature. These are:

- Electronic searching using computer-held databases
- Searching reference lists of articles you already have
- Hand searching relevant journals specific to the research topic or using electronic journal searching
- Contacting authors directly
- Searching national guidelines/professional body sites.

Computer held databases

Searching for literature has become a far easier and efficient process with the advent of electronic databases for literature searching.

If you have recently visited your local academic library, you will be very aware that the computer revolution has had a large impact on the ways in which we search for information. In the past (when we were students) those reviewing the literature would have to search through hard-bound volumes of subject indexed references in which previously published literature was categorised under various keywords. They could not be immediately updated and updates took place often on a yearly basis. Those seeking information had no alternative other than to trawl through bound volumes to find information on a topic or by an author (and then commonly, anything published within the last year was unobtainable because it was in the process of binding). Nowadays, all the information you need is accessible through one of many databases.

What are databases?

In general there are two types of database.

- **Subject specific databases** (e.g. MEDLINE) contain references for your topic of interest and allows you to search for that information, normally in the form of published academic papers (journal articles). These databases are compiled as follows: published papers are scrutinised and allocated keywords which are then indexed. This index of keywords is then stored by the database. When you come to search the database, you enter a keyword and the database produces a list of references of the papers it holds which have been allocated your keyword. Normally, the reference is given in the form of name, date of publication, title of publication, title of journal in which the information is held and possibly an abstract for the paper.
- **Electronic journal databases**. This is useful when you know exactly what you are looking for and have a reference for a particular journal article. You can locate the journal you need and from that you can locate the particular article you need to get hold of . . . It is usually organised via an A–Z section which contains access to the electronic copy of the papers (journal articles). It is important to note that the electronic journal database does not allow you to search for what is written on your topic (the subject specific database is better for this) but is useful to locate the sources identified from the subject specific databases.

If you are serious about searching for the best available information or evidence, then you are advised to contact your local subject librarian for a tutorial on how to use the relevant databases. You will need to be familiar with the passwords required to access them and this can avert the frustrating process of not being able to access the databases you require. In some cases searching on-site in your university or place of work is easier than doing it from home.

Getting started using databases

- Identify databases to which you have access and to establish the relevance of these.
  - Various health and social care databases will be available through professional websites, university or organisational libraries to which you belong.
  - Different databases access literature from different countries or groups of countries or focus on specific specialities or interest areas. You need to ensure you use an appropriate one.
- Find out if you need a password to access these and set one up. Your librarian will help with this.
- Familiarise yourself with the way in which this database works and do note that all databases operate differently – do not assume that commands you use for one database will be understood by another.

Commonly held databases include:

Allied and Alternative Medicine (AMED): Allied and Complementary Medicine is a unique database covering the fields of complementary or alternative medicine.

Applied Social Sciences Index and Abstracts (ASSIA): an indexing and abstracting tool covering health, social services, psychology, sociology, economics, politics, race relations and education.

British Nursing Index (BNI): contains references to British based nursing and midwifery journal articles.

Cochrane Library: database holding systematic reviews for health and social care.

Cumulative Index to Nursing and Allied Health Literature (CINAHL): American based resource for nursing and allied health literature.

Dissertation Abstracts: a definitive subject, title and author guide to virtually every American dissertation accepted at an accredited institution since 1861.

Index to Theses: a comprehensive listing of theses with abstracts accepted for higher degrees by universities in Great Britain and Ireland since 1716.

Medline: broad database covering all areas of medicine and professions allied to medicine.

PsycINFO: is an abstract database of psychological literature from the 1800s to the present.

Social Care Online: open access database for social care journal articles, websites and government publications.

Social Services Abstracts: abstracts of journal articles, dissertations, book reviews.

Sociofile: sociological abstracts/abstracts of journal articles on theoretical and applied sociology.

System for Information on Grey Literature in Europe: a bibliographic database holding non-conventional literature (so called grey literature) in pure and applied natural sciences, and social sciences.

Web of Science: includes science citation index and social science citation index.

Searching electronic databases

We would like to emphasise that the process of searching each of these databases will vary from one to another and you are advised to seek appropriate assistance from your academic/professional subject librarian to do so. You may find it useful to use a table such as the one below which helps with the following PICOT question.

The general principles are as follows:

Make sure you make use of the AND/OR commands in the searching strategy as appropriate.

AND ensures that **each** term you have entered is searched for. This will reduce the number of hits you get as each term must be included in the article for it to be recognised.

OR ensures that **either one term or another** is selected. This will increase the number of hits you get as you only need to identify one of the terms for the article to be selected.

If you keep getting results that are not useful you may wish to use **NOT** to **exclude** specific topics

The use of AND, OR and NOT are called **Boolean operators**.

 There is also the *** facility** which enables you to identify all possible endings of the key term you write. You need to identify the 'root' of the word for example, the part of the word that doesn't change – and put the * after that last letter.

Example: child* will identify articles containing child, children, children's and so on.

Example question: What is the **attitude** of **student** (nurse or other **profession**) to **HIV/AIDS**?

	1 Keyword		2 Keyword		3 Keyword		4 Keyword
a)	Attitude*	AND	Student*	AND	Nurse (or state other profession)	AND	Human immunodeficiency virus
	or		or		or		or
b)	Stigma		Baccalaureate*		Nurs*		HIV
	or		or				or
c)	Approach*		Undergraduate*				H.I.V.
	or		or				or
d)	Opinion*		Pre-registration				Acquired immuno-deficiency syndrome
	or		or				or
e)	View*		Pre-qualifying				AIDS

adapted from Oldershaw (2009)

Activity: Try and identify search terms for a question you have using this table (you can add rows or columns as you need to). Column 5 may be used to record the number of hits (or results).

	1 Keyword		2 Keyword		3 Keyword		4 Keyword	5 No. of hits
	or	AND	or	AND	or	AND	or	
	or		or		or		or	
	or		or		or		or	

You can also specify whether you would like to search throughout **the whole article** for the term, or whether you are going to limit your search to the **abstract** (the short summary) or **title**.

- If you limit your search to the identification of the term in just the title, you will exclude a lot of references which might be relevant to you, as some titles will not use the key terms you have identified.
- If you search through the whole articles for your keyword, you are likely to be overwhelmed with literature.
- Limiting your search to the abstract is likely to be a suitable compromise.
- If you get few articles on a less common or unusual keyword you may want to search in the whole article.

You are likely to need to refine your searching strategy as you progress. You will find that you will develop new ideas as you undertake the searching process. You might find, for example, a key theme is called by a different name or phrase that you had not previously thought of. Be aware of this and be prepared to search using new and different terms.

Once you have identified the key literature on your topic using one database, you could repeat the search using another database. This will depend on the requirements of your search. If you find that the same references are thrown up, then you can be confident that your strategy is well focussed and that you are accessing the relevant literature on your topic. You might feel it is appropriate to scale down your search.

Remember . . .

- Searching for literature is time consuming and needs skill – you are advised not to leave it until the last minute before searching.
- If you do not have any 'hits' from your search, then you need to keep searching with different keywords until you identify literature which is linked to your topic area. If you have too many hits, you will need to refocus your search.
- Remember to keep a record of the search terms you have used and the results of these searches.

If new references are constantly being thrown up, you will need to continue searching until later searches reveal little or no new information.

Why is electronic searching not 100% effective?

Despite the advances in electronic searching, computerised searching tools are not 100% effective and will fail to identify some of the relevant literature on your topic.

This is because:

- Some relevant literature might have been categorised using different keywords and would therefore not be identified by one particular search strategy.

- The topic you are looking for may be mentioned in several papers but not to a large extent and therefore is not indexed when these papers are entered onto the database. This means that the papers will not be recognised by the databases when you search for this topic.
- You may have only searched within the title of articles.
- The title may be misleading.

Hawker *et al.* (2002) identify how authors who use humorous titles for their work run the risk that their work will not be identified by those who search on the topic. Although using various keywords will help identify literature that is not identified on the first search, it is still possible for literature to remain unidentified even though it is highly relevant to addressing the research question.

Is searching for evidence an art or a science?

We have emphasised that searching for evidence will never be a one-off process. You will need to ensure you have strived for a thorough coverage of the available evidence and continue to update and refine your searches. The more you search, the more you will begin to develop instinct and experience about where to search and what terms are used around your subject matter. Knowledge of your subject matter will certainly help with this.

Example: an inexperienced searcher may search for 'use of gloves AND aprons' in infection control. A more experienced individual will recognise that it may be better to search under the terms 'universal OR standard precautions' rather than seek out the individual protective equipment.

Therefore, you should regard searching for evidence as both a science and an art. Searching should be regarded as a science, because we encourage you to undertake a methodological and comprehensive approach to the identification of relevant evidence. Searching should also be regarded as an art because you also need to be creative and flexible about the way you identify relevant evidence.

Searching the reference lists

Once you have identified the key articles that relate to your research question, you might want to scrutinise the reference lists of those **key articles** for further references that may be useful to you. You will use the same keywords and inclusion and exclusion criteria to do this, although you may come across older key texts, which are frequently referenced, but that fall outside your exclusion dates.

Hand-searching relevant journals

If you have been able to identify that many of your key articles which are relevant to your research question are located in one or two journals, it might be useful to hand-search these journals to see whether you can identify other relevant articles that have not been identified through other searching strategies. Searching through the contents pages of these journals may identify other relevant material. This may also be done electronically through A–Z of journals and selecting the relevant journal (some journal websites have archive search facilities).

Author searching/using experts

If you find that many of your key articles are by the same author(s) then it may be useful to carry out an author search in order to identify whether the author(s) have published other work which has not been identified in the electronic search. This might also lead you towards work in progress. In some specialist areas it may be worth contacting the author directly to see if they are aware of any other sources.

Experts in a clinical or professional area may have attended conferences or be involved in projects that address your issue or question. Contacting them directly may highlight new sources. If they have been helpful, it is considered polite to share your findings with them once your research is complete. If your topic includes a product or service then the manufacturers/suppliers may have commissioned research. You need to be aware of the potential bias of such research.

Grey literature

Grey literature is a term used to describe literature that has not been published and is therefore hard to find. If the area is under-researched, you might find that useful grey literature does exist. You can identify this literature in a number of ways, such as contacting known authors in an area and asking if they know of other sources of information. However, use of grey literature is unlikely to be a main component of your literature search.

Publications of professional bodies

Remember that your professional body will have many resources and it will be useful to look at these to find additional sources of information.

A **combination of these searching strategies** will ensure that you have the most comprehensive search strategy and therefore the most chance of retrieving the information that is relevant to your research question. However, you can never be certain that you have obtained all the literature on a particular topic. Greenhalgh and Peacock (2005) refer to this process as **'snowball sampling'** where you are pointed in the direction of additional literature from your existing literature. For example, if useful articles are found in a particular journal, then this journal is further scrutinised for other relevant material. This strategy cannot be pre-specified and is dependent on the results of early literature searching.

It is recommended that you avoid statements in your writing that declare that there is **no literature** on a particular topic and state instead, if asked, that **no** literature *was identified* on the topic in question.

How to use abstracts to confirm the relevance of the paper

Once you have identified the literature that is relevant to you, the next step is to sort through the reference list you now have and identify which references are most relevant. To do this, you cannot rely on the title alone. This is because the focus of the article, whether or not it is a primary research study, is often unclear from the title alone.

Rather than rely on the title to determine the relevance of a paper to your research question, it is preferable to read the **abstract** for each reference you have identified.

The abstract will give you a summary of the content of the article, in particular whether it is a research article or not.

The abstract is often available on the electronic databases such as CINAHL or MEDLINE. However, abstracts can themselves be unreliable sources for determining the exact focus of a paper, and you might find that you miss relevant literature if you discard a paper because of the information contained in the abstract. However, given that you are unlikely to be able to access in full each paper you identify from an electronic search, it is likely that you will have to rely on the abstract to determine whether or not you include a paper to address your research question. You can document this if you write up the limitations of the approach you have taken.

- Once you have accessed the abstracts for your references, refer back to the inclusion and exclusion criteria you have set for yourself and assess each of the abstracts according to the perceived relevance for your question.
- You can then determine which references meet your criteria and which do not. Retain those which do and discard those which clearly do not.
- If you cannot tell from the abstract, you will need to access the paper in order to do this.
- By undertaking this process, you should be able to edit your reference lists

to those articles and information which are directly relevant to your research question.

- You can now use this edited reference list to locate the articles that are relevant to your research question.

Getting hold of your sources from the references

The references to which you are directed are likely to be found in journals, books and other publications.

 Activity: Try and get training on using your local library (especially from a subject specialist) to help you locate publications.

- Most university and workplace libraries will have many journals accessible as '**full-text**' electronically and you will find that you can locate and download many articles without leaving your computer. **You will need a password to access these**. There is sometimes – but not always – a link from the database to the full text article in the electronic library.
- You are strongly advised to familiarise yourself with the journals to which you have easy access through your local library. Some libraries will have a subject specific catalogue.
- If the reference you require is not available full-text electronically, then you will need to access the bound volumes which are available as hard copies in the library.
- If the references are not available electronically or in bound volumes in your local library, then you will need to either arrange to visit another library or arrange an **inter-library loan**. This will have a small cost and be time consuming so you will need to make a decision about the effort you go to.
- It may be worth trying a general internet search for the article as increasingly articles are posted on websites. Do make sure it is the complete original article (best as a pdf file) and that it has not been summarised or altered.

Strengths and limitations of your searching strategy

Clearly, those doing a more detailed systematic review need to make every effort to retrieve the articles relevant to their study. Those undertaking a smaller scale literature search do not need to go to the same lengths to retrieve literature, although of course the more comprehensive the search, the better. Overall, your search will be more comprehensive the more effort you make in locating all the references that are central to your question.

Some potential limitations of a search

Experience of the researchers

If you are doing a project by yourself, you are unlikely to have the same resources as a team of people working together. Those working together can share ideas, read abstracts and papers together and so on. If you are a novice researcher you are more likely to miss sources than a more experienced searcher.

Potential bias

You should identify any potential bias of the sources you used – if you have been unable to track down certain sources, you should acknowledge this. If you have limited your sources by accessibility then this is a limitation or if papers you find are sponsored by companies or organisations that may influence the results this should be recognised.

5. Recording your searching strategy

Consider how you are going to manage and store the references you identify. Think about the method that suits you best in terms of keeping track of references and maintain it.

It may be helpful to keep a record of your searching strategy, the keywords that you used and the number of hits so that you can demonstrate a systematic approach.

See the table earlier in this chapter and consider using one of the columns to record the number of hits. This may be of particular use for academic assignments or if you are sharing the results of your search with other professionals/ colleagues as evidence for your practice. The reader should clearly be able to see how you refined your search and got to the final ones that you reviewed.

Example: If you are searching for primary research articles concerned with smoking and social care, you might initially undertake two basic searches and then combine these searches:

> Databases: CINAHL 1994 – Search term: smok*: Total number of hits: 30,000
>
> Databases: CINAHL 1994 – Search term: smok* AND social care* Total number of hits: 15,000

You can then demonstrate how you combined this search with another search in order to obtain a more manageable number of hits.

It might also be useful to demonstrate the success of your searching strategy and which searches yielded the best results. It is also useful to state what type of literature your hits included, if you can determine this from the abstract available. If you are searching for articles of primary research but are failing to identify these, you can document this.

Tips for documenting your search strategy

- Remember that the aim is to demonstrate how you undertook a systematic approach to your searching.
- Discuss the approach you took to develop effective search strategies.
- Keep a record of all the search terms used so that you can provide evidence of your approach if asked.
- Keep a record of the other approaches you employed to search for literature.
- Be able to comment on the effectiveness of the approaches you used. For example, if electronic searching did not yield as many hits as you had hoped, discuss why this might have been.
- Make every effort to obtain relevant literature.
- It is more accurate to write 'I did not find any literature on X' rather than categorically 'there is no literature . . .'

6. Manage and store your literature effectively

Remember to:

- Back up (save) all your records and keep them in a safe place throughout your searching process.
- Keep records on more than one site (what if your computer was stolen or there was a fire?) consider emailing a copy of your reference list to yourself.
- If you are using full text electronic copies of articles then set up a folder so they are all together.
- Write references down in full every time you read something useful. It is very frustrating to have to track down page numbers or editions of references you have mislaid.
- Some people choose to keep a card filing system for all references.
- Consider using a reference manager such as ENDNOTE which will hold all your references electronically and produce a reference list in the format you require.
- A clear record should show how you got to the articles you are using to

underpin your conclusions and so it could be repeated by someone else who would identify the same articles.

In summary

You should by now be well aware of the importance of a systematic search strategy. This will ensure that you access a comprehensive range of literature that is relevant to your question. The use of inclusion and exclusion criteria can be very useful in ensuring that the literature identified is relevant to your review question. The need to combine the electronic searching of relevant databases with additional strategies such as hand-searching journals and reference lists has been discussed. You need to be aware that electronic searching can never be fully comprehensive and that 'snowball sampling', using many different strategies to identify literature will usually be the most effective way of achieving the most comprehensive literature search. At the end of the searching process, you will achieve a list of references that are relevant to your research question which you will be able to locate in your academic/ professional library.

At this point, you should be confident that you have identified the most relevant literature that will enable you to answer your research question. You should be aware of the strengths and limitations of your search strategy and be prepared to justify your approach if asked. It is now time to stand back and take a critical look at the literature you have identified. We will discuss how you do this in the next chapter.

Key points

1 You need a focussed question in order to identify your search terms.
2 It is important to identify the types of literature that will enable you to answer your research question.
3 Inclusion and exclusion criteria should be specific to your question.
4 The literature search strategy should incorporate a variety of approaches including electronic searching, hand searching and reference list searching.
5 The limitations of these approaches should be acknowledged.

6

How do I know if the evidence is convincing and useful?

Defining the terms • Getting to know your literature • What is critical appraisal? • The importance of critical appraisal • Getting started with critical appraisal • Useful websites for critical appraisal • Key questions to ask when critically appraising ALL pieces of evidence • Key questions to ask of review articles • Example of critical appraisal tools of review articles • Key questions to ask of quantitative studies • How should we critique qualitative research? • Example of critical appraisal tools for non-research papers • Incorporating critical appraisal into your academic writing and in practice • In summary • Key points

In this chapter we will explore how you can tell if the information and evidence you find is any good or not. Overall we want you to move from a position where you would be tempted to say *'I've read this so it must be true'* to a position where you say *'I've read this – now I need to know if it is reliable'*. Specifically we will explore:

- How to judge the quality and quantity of evidence we use (critical appraisal)
- How to assess the influence of one article
- How to identify what is important in different sources of evidence including expert opinion and websites
- How to use a simple appraisal tool.

Every time you read the newspapers you probably form a judgement of whether or not you believe what you read; you might even wonder which sources were used to write the article. If you don't believe what you read, you might be tempted to track down the source upon which the article is based. Then what usually happens (well, for us anyway) is that you don't have time to research this further and you never really find out if what you read is true or not . . . Now consider the way you approach your professional reading. Just as we are sceptical about what we read in the papers, so we should be about what we read in the academic journals.

Activity: Access some research from a professional journal and see if you can identify critical comment on the paper. Many journals offer a review of the paper along side the article or in the next edition. Try and spot how a reviewer offers both positive and negative comment on the paper.

Refer back to how you have used literature in the past and consider the potential problems with your approach. Did you:

- Scan read it?
- Use only one or two sources?
- Only use what agreed with the point you wanted to make?
- Only use readily available sources?
- Ignored research that didn't agree with your current practice?
- Just use quotes or sections that agree with your view?
- Believe everything that is written without questioning the authority of the writer or the quality of the arguments or evidence?

Defining the terms

When you are reading about evaluating the evidence, you will find that many phrases come up time and time again. It is important to know what we mean by these phrases.

- **Rigour** – is the research credible and believable, usually relating to thoroughness of approach to the research?
- **Validity** – does it accurately measure/report what it says it does?
- **Reliability** – would the same results/conclusions be found if the research was repeated?

- **Relevance** – does it apply to my client group and context?
- **Credibility** – is there evidence that the results or conclusions are believable?

In addition:

- **Strengths** – refer to the good things about the literature, in relation to the points above.
- **Limitations** – refer to what could be criticised about the literature, in relation to the points above.

Getting to know your literature

The first thing to do when getting started with evaluating your evidence is to become familiar with the literature you have got.

- **Read** and **re-read** the material so that you become familiar with it. At this point, you should be able to discuss with confidence the content of your research papers and be able to identify what type of evidence you have.
- Study carefully the research methods used in each research paper that you have. **Make sure you understand them**.
- Begin to determine the strengths, limitations and relevance of the information to the question you need to address.
- At first glance, a research paper might appear to address your research question directly, however on closer inspection you realise that the scope of the paper is very different from what your initial assessment had led you to believe and in fact has only indirect relevance to your research question.
- You might find that although the context of the paper is relevant to your research question, the methods used in the paper have been poorly carried out and you are less confident in the results of the study as a result.

Making sense of each individual research paper you come across is therefore very important and will enable you to make important assessments as to the relevance of the paper to your topic of study in addition to identifying the strengths and limitations – and therefore the impact – that the paper will have on addressing what you are trying to find out.

What is critical appraisal?

Critical appraisal is the structured process of examining a piece of research in order to **determine its strengths and limitations** and therefore the **relevance or weight** it should have in addressing your research question.

In essence you are **evaluating or judging the quality and usefulness** of the evidence you have.

There is a useful guide to critical appraisal in the 'what is' series (Burls 2009) www.whatisseries.co.uk/whatis/pdfs/what_is_crit_appr.pdf

The importance of critical appraisal

The controversy surrounding the measles, mumps and rubella (MMR) vaccination described in Chapter 4 illustrates the importance of undertaking critical appraisal of all research and other information that you encounter. Any practitioner who had read Wakefield's original article could see at a glance that the evidence it provided was not strong evidence – yet a media scare took over and there was evidence that both practitioners become reluctant to administer the MMR vaccination and parents became reluctant to take their children for vaccination. The MMR controversy illustrates the importance of critical appraisal of research and other information so that you can identify how strong and relevant the evidence is relating to a particular topic.

If you are new to evaluating the literature, you might fall into one of two categories:

1 **You accept any piece of research** or other information at face value and accept what is written without question. You may believe that a paper published in a high quality journal or written by an expert is above critique and so do not attempt any structured appraisal of the paper. Even a paper that is published in a reputable journal must be examined for validity and the relevance that it has to the topic area.
2 You may interpret the term 'critical appraisal' to mean that **you must criticise and find fault** with everything that you read. Often the term critical is interpreted to mean that unless you 'tear to pieces' what you find, then you have not done your job. Although it is always possible to find faults with every piece of research, it needs to be remembered that no research is perfect. Therefore when you look for strengths and weaknesses remember to take a balanced approach. More credible authors may identify

within their own methodology what they consider to be any weaknesses with their approach.

Getting started with critical appraisal

The first step in the critical appraisal process is to identify what type of information you have. Start getting to know your literature. At this point it is normal to feel swamped by the amount of literature.

 Activity: you may want to organise a table or index cards to help you sort out the information you have. Consider using colour highlighters or Post-it notes to help with this.

Identify what types of evidence you have

You are advised to collect your references together and identify what is a literature review, a research paper, a discussion paper or other information. You will have already worked out the type of evidence you need to answer your question and you need to be clear what types of literature you have.

- Overall, you will probably have a combination of qualitative and quantitative research, maybe some systematic reviews and other non-research information, such as discussion and opinion articles.
- Group your literature together so that you have all the qualitative research papers in one pile, the quantitative papers in another, discussion and opinion in another and so on.
- When you have done this, you will be able to identify the types of literature you have and you will then be able to think carefully about how you will appraise the literature that you have.

As discussed above you will have read each paper several times until you can summarise what is going on in each paper.

- **Research papers** (including **literature reviews or systematic reviews**) normally begin with a specific **research question** which is addressed using an identified **method**, following which the **results, discussion** and **conclusions** are presented.
- **Discussion or opinion papers** will not have this structure and will be introduced as representing the opinion of the author. Remember that the quality of this type of evidence will depend on the person writing the paper but remember also not to assume that an expert is using relevant evidence

based sources upon which he bases his argument. There may be bias in the selection of the sources used.

- **Paper giving general information/updates about a topic.** It can be confusing to identify whether such updates have been compiled using a systematic process or not. In principle, if the paper does not include a specific question and a method recounting how the update was put together, you should not consider this to be a comprehensive review. This will provide less strong evidence than a review which has been compiled systematically.

It is important to note that the first step in critical appraisal is getting to know your literature. Using a critical appraisal tool (which we will describe later) will not help you much, if you do not understand the basic principles of the research design of the study you are critiquing.

Ask yourself why the study was undertaken or why the paper was written. Then if the paper reports a research study how the study was conducted and what the main results were.

You need to be familiar with all the material that you have before you can move on to more detailed critical appraisal. It is always a good test of how well you know the literature if you can discuss the literature you have found in detail with someone else without referring back to the papers or at least with minimal reference!

Once you have become familiar with your literature, the next step is to decide how you will critically appraise the literature that you have.

Critical appraisal tools

Critical appraisal tools are **checklists** to help you ask questions of the evidence you have in order to assist you in determining **how strong** and **how relevant** the evidence is.

Simply put you are trying to find out if it is worth your while looking at the study, what are the results and whether the results are relevant to your practice.

- Critical appraisal tools help you develop a consistent approach to the critique of research and other information.
- However they only help with the critical appraisal – they do not do the work for you! If you do not understand the methods by which the research has been undertaken, the tool will not help you. Therefore you need to understand what is going on in the paper before you begin to appraise it.

Benefits of using an appraisal tool

- The review process is complex and use of an appraisal tool will assist in the development of a systematic approach to this process and to ensure that all papers are reviewed with equal rigour.
- They will guide you through questions you need to ask of each type of paper you have.

Which appraisal tool should I use?

There are a vast number of critical appraisal tools available. A quick search engine search (such as Google) will enable you to identify a good many, others can be found in research or study skills textbooks.

 It is probably most useful to use an **appraisal tool** that is relevant to the type of research you are using and that helps you to evaluate the usefulness and relevance of your papers; however, this is not always possible.

You will find generic appraisal tools which you can use on all types of evidence, tools that have been developed for use on all types of research and tolls that are specific to one type of research.

General critical appraisal tools

If you are new to critical appraisal and are looking for a general checklist to help you evaluate the evidence you come across, Cottrell (2005) has developed a generic appraisal tool which you can use to evaluate any piece of academic writing. This is a relatively straightforward tool to use and is a good start if you are new to critical appraisal.

Other generic tools are available in many research textbooks, for example *Essentials of Nursing Research* by Polit and Beck (2005). Most of the critical appraisal tools that you encounter are designed to appraise empirical research. Tools and assessment strategies are also available for assessing the quality of published material that does not fall under the category of empirical research, but these are less well developed. Methods for approaching the critical appraisal of **non-research papers** are discussed at the end of the chapter.

You might also find the following series of papers in the *British Medical Journal* useful. They can of course be accessed electronically.

Specific critical appraisal tools

For those who have already had some experience of critical appraisal, you might want to start with the more specific critical appraisal tools which focus on a specific research methodology. Appraisal tools which are specifically focussed on the type of research paper you have will contain questions which are closely related to the specific study design in question, providing an appropriate structure for the review. Many critical appraisal tools have been developed for the review of specific types of research, and as such are design specific, for example, for the review of randomised controlled trials only.

For example, the University of Oxford Public Health Resources Unit have developed a series of critical appraisal tools. The Critical Appraisal Skills Programme (CASP) has produced critical appraisal tools for the appraisal of many different types of research including randomised controlled trials, systematic reviews, cohort and case control studies and qualitative studies. The advantage of the CASP critical appraisal tools is that there is a specific critical appraisal tools for most common types of studies you are likely to encounter.

The **Critical Appraisal Skills Programme (CASP)** critical appraisal tools are available at: http://www.phru.nhs.uk/Pages/PHD/resources.htm and there are different tools for different types of research.

As a novice appraiser and at undergraduate level, you are advised to consider the ten main questions only and not to consider the additional more detailed questions. Those studying at postgraduate level might want to refer to these more detailed questions.

Other websites offer a variety of specific tools and you may want to consider if any of your own professional journals relating to evidence based practice offer tools.

Useful websites for critical appraisal

Therapy and prevention http://www.cche.net/principles/content_therapy.asp

Diagnosis http://www.cche.net/principles/content_diagnosis.asp

Harm http://www.cche.net/principles/content_harm.asp

Prognosis http://www.cche.net/principles/content_prognosis.asp

Overview articles http://www.cche.net/principles/content_overview.asp

Clinical decision analyses http://www.cche.net/principles/content_d_analysis.asp

Clinical practice guidelines http://www.cche.net/principles/ content_p_guideline.asp

Clinical utilisation reviews* http://www.cche.net/principles/ content_u_review.asp

Outcomes of health service research: http://www.cche.net/principles/ content_v_outcome.asp

Quality of life measures http://www.cche.net/principles/content_qol.asp

Economic analyses http://www.cche.net/principles/content_e_analysis.asp

Grading Healthcare Recommendations http://www.cche.net/principles/ content_grading.asp

Applicability of clinical trials results http://www.cche.net/principles/ content_results.asp

Probability for different diagnoses http://www.cche.net/principles/ content_d_probability.asp

 Activity: Refer back to Chapter 4 in this book or access a research textbook to find out more about the research methods that are used in the papers you have accessed.

If you come across lots of different types of evidence using different research methodologies, then this is harder to make sense of because you need to understand all the different approaches used. Clearly this is harder if your literature search leads you to a wide cross-section of research methods as this will lead you to many different research approaches.

Key questions to ask when critically appraising ALL pieces of evidence

The following questions should be asked of all research papers:

Q. What is the journal of publication?
You should be aware of the quality of the journal in which the research is published.

- In principle, a journal is considered to be of good quality if it is **peer reviewed** – that is, each paper is reviewed by at least one recognised expert in the subject area about which the paper is written prior to acceptance for publication in the journal.
- However it should be noted that the peer review process is not perfect. Papers are generally considered by one or two experts in a field and it is not possible for an expert to know every aspect about any particular topic.
- It is not uncommon for corrections or amendments to a paper to appear in later publications of the journal. In reality, the peer review process takes place when the research paper is published!
- As a general rule, just as you may be more likely to take an argument more seriously if it is published in one newspaper than another, this is also the case with academic journals.

Q. Who wrote the paper?

In all the literature you encounter, it is particularly important that the researchers have the necessary experience to undertake the research or the authority to write the article. Some people argue that this is especially import-ant in qualitative research as the quality of the data collected is dependent on the skills of the researcher. Their own values, experience and interests shape the research process.

Therefore, questions that can be asked about the author include:

- What are their qualifications and are they relevant to the question?
- What is their experience and is it relevant to the question they ask?
- Do they have the necessary insight into the topic area to address the research question?

Access a journal's website for an overview of its publishing process and ask educationalists/senior colleagues what are considered high quality journals in your profession.

Q. What is the purpose of the evidence/research paper?

You need to establish this first of all so that you can determine how you will evaluate the paper. If it is a research paper, the study question should be clear and should be founded on argument and rationale as to why the study was undertaken. If it is a discussion paper, the authors should state this early on in the paper.

We will now discuss the **key questions** you should ask of the different types of evidence you are likely to encounter and provide some examples of critical appraisal tools you might find useful.

- Review articles
- Quantitative studies

- Qualitative studies
- Professional and clinical guidelines and policy
- Non-research information, for example discussion and opinion or anecdotal evidence
- Websites.

Key questions to ask of review articles

Q. Has the review been undertaken systematically?
Those evaluating review articles should be able to determine whether the review was undertaken in an explicit systematic way or whether a more narrative approach has been used.

Q. Are the researchers explicit about the methods used to achieve this review?
A review incorporating a systematic approach will present stronger evidence than a review in which the method is not explicit. The amount of detail given to the search, critiquing and bringing together of the evidence will differ with each literature review. You should scrutinise the methods used to conduct the review.

Q. Do the researchers demonstrate that they did everything in their power to ensure their approach was as systematic as possible?
If the review is described as a **Cochrane Collaboration review** you can be fairly confident that it is a review that has been undertaken systematically.

A **less detailed review** is likely to be carried out by a single researcher with fewer resources for collaboration in these aspects. A less detailed review acknowledges that the search will not be comprehensive but will **identify which databases were searched**.

Example: a Cochrane-style systematic review aims to uncover **all literature** on the topic in question. it will have a team of researchers who work together in the critical analysis of the literature,

See if you can find a review article relating to your profession using a database or from the Cochrane website www.cochrane.org

Example of critical appraisal tools of review articles

One of the critical appraisal tools for the appraisal of a systematic review is the CASP tool for systematic reviews available at: http://www.phru.nhs.uk/ Doc_Links/S.Reviews%20Appraisal%20Tool.pdf

Crombie (2006) discusses the critical appraisal of review papers and suggests that those undertaking a critical appraisal of a review should consider the following essential questions:

- How were the papers identified?
- How was the quality of the papers assessed?
- How were the results summarised?

Greenhalgh's paper (1997a) entitled 'Papers that summarise other papers (systematic reviews and meta-analyses)' is a useful reference here and incorporates a 'how to' guide for appraising a review. This paper can be accessed electronically at http://www.bmj.com/cgi/content/full/315/7109/672

Key questions to ask of quantitative studies

Most quantitative studies that you will encounter fall into one of the following categories:

- Randomised controlled trial (or similar trial)
- Case control study
- Cohort study
- Cross-sectional studies using questionnaire/surveys.

One of the main approaches to assessing the quality of quantitative work is to assess the validity and reliability of the study.

- **Validity** refers to whether the study measures what it intends to measure.
- **Reliability** refers to whether the measurement is reliable and would yield the same results on repeated measurements.

Using a database, see if you can find a quantitative study relating to your profession.

Q. What method was selected to undertake the research?
In most papers there will be a short summary of the research process under-taken and from this you will be able to identify how the study was conducted.

Q. How big was the sample?
The sample refers to those who took part in the study.

The authors of quantitative research papers should demonstrate how they determined the sample size for the research in question. This should be clearly documented in the paper and is often referred to as a **power calculation**. The power calculation is a statistical test undertaken by those designing the research study in order to ensure that the sample used in the research is big enough for the findings to be considered reliable. For example, the findings of a small study are likely to be less reliable than those of a larger study as they may be due to chance variations. With a larger sample, the findings are less likely to be due to chance. A power calculation is undertaken to determine the number of participants needed to undertake a study in order to obtain reliable findings.

Q. Has the appropriate sample been obtained?
You need to ask yourself, who was selected to participate in the study? Quanti-tative research sometimes uses **random sampling**. This means that the sample is picked at random from the overall population.

When you are reviewing a quantitative study, be aware of the sampling strategy and be able to comment on the reasons as to why this approach has been adopted. Consider whether a random or non-random sample was used and whether this was appropriate.

Q. How were the data collected?
The data collection method should be appropriate for the study design. Quanti-tative research often uses a wide range of data collection methods that are appropriate for objective measurement such as survey/questionnaires, object-ive physiological tests, observation, and rates of occurrence (incidence).

Q. How were the data analysed?
Quantitative data are usually analysed statistically and you should expect to find reference to the statistical tests used in the paper in order to make sense of the data. The data should be clearly described so that you can identify the main findings of the paper.

Additional resources for those reviewing RCTs

In addition to the specific CASP appraisal tools, there are further resources for those reviewing quantitative studies. The CONSORT (Consolidated Standards of Reporting Trials 2001) have produced the **CONSORT Statement** available at http://www.consort-statement.org/ which is an evidence-based, minimum set of recommendations for reporting RCTs. It offers a standard way for authors to prepare reports of trial findings, facilitating their complete and transparent reporting, and aiding their critical appraisal and interpretation. Full details of the revised CONSORT statement are given by Moher *et al.* (2001). The statement includes discussion of the scientific background for the study, eligibility of participants and interventions intended for each group, random allocation and blinding, statistical analysis and discussion of results.

Additional key questions and resources for those reviewing cohort studies

Rochon *et al.* (2005) have identified factors to consider when considering the quality of the studies. These can be used in conjunction with the CASP critical appraisal tool for cohort studies.

Q How were the groups selected and how were they defined?
The important difference between an RCT and a cohort study is that in an RCT there are two or more groups that are allocated at random. In a cohort study, the cohort and control group are not allocated at random but arise naturally in the population.

Q. Does the comparison makes sense? In other words was a cohort study a useful method of studying the research topic?
There must be an obvious comparison group in a cohort study.

Example: those who use illicit drugs might be a naturally occurring cohort group. This group of illicit drug users can then be compared with non-users. Any differences between the two groups cannot be attributed to the exposure or intervention given as the cohort and control groups were never equal.

Additional key questions and resources for those reviewing case control studies

Crombie (2006) suggests that the following essential questions are asked of case control studies:

Q. How were the cases obtained?
Q. Was the control group appropriate?
Q. Was data collected in the same way for cases as for controls?

Additional key questions and resources for those reviewing survey/questionnaires

Boynton and Greenhalgh (2004 p.1312) assert: 'No single method has been so abused.' They also warn that elementary errors in carrying out questionnaire or survey research are common. Therefore you should proceed with your appraisal of questionnaires with care! In addition, there is a lack of formal appraisal tools or checklists to assist with the process of critical appraisal. Boynton and Greenhalgh suggest the following questions to appraise the studies:

Q. What information is required and is a questionnaire appropriate?
You need to consider whether a questionnaire is the most appropriate way of collecting data for the study in question.

Q. Is there an existing instrument and has it has been tested for validity and reliability?
Using an existing questionnaire which has been rigorously tested (also known as piloted or validated) to check that it asks the right questions in a clear way is vital. If the questionnaire has not been tested out in this way the data might not be worth the paper it is written on!

Q. How was the sample selected?
The researchers should justify why they picked the sample group that they did and why it is appropriate to the study.

Q. How many people responded to the questionnaire?
This is another vital question. If you only get 20% responding, what about the 80% you do not know about. There might be something very different about the 20% who responded compared to the 80% who did not.

Can you think of when you have found a questionnaire hard to answer or when the meaning of the questions has been unclear?

Overall, for those critiquing quantitative research, there are two main objectives.

• You should become as familiar as possible with the research approach undertaken in the study.
• You should apply this knowledge when reviewing the rigour of the study with the use of an appropriate critical appraisal tool.

The next time you find a questionnaire, or are asked to complete one, try and critically appraise it using some of the principles outlined above.

An example of critical appraisal tools for quantitative research are the CASP guidelines which have tools for reviewing randomised controlled trials, cohort studies, case control studies.

Key questions to ask of qualitative studies

There has been much discussion in recent years concerning the ways in which qualitative research is evaluated and this debate is ongoing. This is because there is often no set approach or standard for carrying out qualitative research and it is therefore difficult to evaluate it.

There has been an increased demand for **evidence of rigour in qualitative research**. Has a thorough and appropriate approach been applied to key research methods in the study? Clearly without evidence of rigour in the undertaking of the study, the worth of any study can be questioned. Because the 'measurements' obtained in qualitative research are made through the interpretation of the researchers, most qualitative researchers argue that it is not possible to assess qualitative research in the same way as quantitative research. For this reason. Lincoln and Guba (1985) argued that the **following terms are more appropriate** to assessing the quality of a qualitative study than terms such as validity and reliability:

- **Credibility** – do the findings ring true from the approach taken? Are they well presented and meaningful?
- **Transferability** – can the results be transferred into a different setting?
- **Dependability** – can you rely on the results as they are presented?
- **Confirmability** – could the study be repeated?

See if you can identify a qualitative research study by accessing a database and looking at the titles and abstracts.

How should we critique qualitative research?

It is important for those who review qualitative research to be aware that there is **no agreement** among qualitative researchers (Popay *et al.* 1998; Sandelowski and Barroso 2002; Russell and Gregory 2003) about:

- What constitutes a good qualitative study
- How a study is critiqued
- What terminology to be used when referring to both qualitative studies and critiquing tools.

They argue that all qualitative researchers should keep an accurate trail of the research process and be transparent in the data analysis process.

Therefore you are likely to encounter a range of qualitative research incorporating different approaches and methods and an equally wide range of appraisal tools for the critique of qualitative research. This means that it can be difficult to determine whether or not the study is any good.

Considering what you know about quantitative and qualitative research what do you think the similarities and differences might be in critical appraisal?

Q. Was the right qualitative research method used?
Refer back to the different approach to qualitative research as outlined in Chapter 4. Then you can ask yourself if the most appropriate approach was used to undertake the study.

Example: researchers who are interested in exploring participants' experience of being homeless might adopt a **phenomenological** approach to their research. It would not be appropriate to observe people who are homeless as this would not achieve an insight into the way in which they would describe their experience. Therefore it is important that the method chosen to address the question is appropriate to the research question itself.

Q. Have the researchers used a qualitative sampling technique?
Appropriate sampling techniques are purposive sampling, theoretical sampling, convenience sampling and snowball sampling. Random sampling would be inappropriate as it may fail to identify information rich participants. The sampling strategy should be justified by the researchers so that you know why they chose the sample they did.

Q. How was the data collected?
The way of collecting the actual data should also be appropriate to the method and research question. The most commonly used data collection methods in qualitative research are

- In-depth interviews
- Focus groups
- Questionnaires may be used for open ended questions
- Observation.

In particular you should be able to identify:

- How the data collection methods were decided upon and whether they are **appropriate** to the research question.
- Is the reason for use of an **in-depth interview** clearly stated? In-depth interviews are used (when the insight into a particular topic is sought from the participant).

- Is the interviewer trained and skilled in asking questions that probe into the experience of the participant and is the aim clearly stated in order to generate rich data through one to one dialogue?

or

- Is the reason for **focus groups** clearly stated? Focus groups are a form of group interview and may be selected over in-depth interviews when dialogue **between research participants** is considered beneficial. If the research topic is unfamiliar to those involved and participants may not have developed their thoughts in relation to this topic, focus groups can be useful as a data collection method as the ideas expressed by one participant may trigger a response in another participant.
- Have the researchers considered the disadvantages (limitations) of the approaches used? **Example:** if a topic is particularly sensitive, participants may be reluctant to express their thoughts in a focus group and in-depth interviews may be more appropriate.

The role of **questionnaires** in the collection of qualitative data should be mentioned at this point. Whilst it is possible to collect qualitative data through open ended questions on a questionnaire schedule, such data is not likely to be as in-depth as that collected through one to one interaction. In particular:

- If **questionnaires** have been used do the researchers recognise that the data may not be as rich as in one to one interviews?
- Do the researchers want to see what people actually do rather than what they say they do? Data collected through **observation** is especially useful for this. **Example:** the extent to which professionals comply with infection control policies can be more accurately measured through direct observation than any other method as it is well known that participants may not accurately self report their behaviour.
- Do the researchers consider the **Hawthorne effect**? The Hawthorne effect refers to the tendency of people who are observed to behave differently (usually better) than they would usually (Eckmanns *et al.* 2006).

It is important to note that observational data may be used in both quantitative and qualitative studies. For example the number of infection control practices undertaken by each practitioner could be counted numerically, or the nature of the interaction between practitioner and patient could be observed using qualitative approaches.

Q. What was the sample for the study and what type of sample was used?
You would expect to see purposive, theoretical, convenience or snowball sampling. Do the researchers give a clear rational for their sampling approach?

What type of participant makes up the purposive sample and are they the most relevant?

Example: if the researchers are exploring people who are homeless, then a purposive sample obtained in one city is likely to be very different to a sample obtained in a different city. Similarly the characteristics of a sample are likely to vary depending on the particular area in the city from which the sample is drawn. This will affect the extent to which the results are transferable from one context to another and therefore the relevance of the particular research study to the literature review question.

Q. How big was the sample?

You would expect the sample size to be large enough to achieve sufficient information rich cases for in-depth data analysis, but not so large that the amount of data obtained becomes unmanageable. Has the way in which the sample size was arrived at been clearly explained?

Q. How were the data collected?

It is important that the researchers justify the approach they have taken to the data collection process and can demonstrate that the process was undertaken systematically and rigorously.

Most researchers agree that in-depth interviews and focus groups should be tape recorded so that the interviews can be **transcribed** (an exact word for word account of what was said). However, some researchers argue that this is time consuming and that the time could be better used by undertaking additional interviews and hence collecting considerably more data.

Q. Was the transcript returned to the participants for validation or not?

There are many variations in the way that qualitative data may be collected. For example, some researchers advocate that interview transcripts are returned to the participants in order that the participants check and **validate** the content of the transcript for accuracy. However, other researchers argue that this is time consuming and unnecessarily burdensome on participants who may not remember the interview or who may not wish to revisit the content of the interview they gave (Barbour 2001). They may also wish to alter the content of the interview, thus affecting its validity.

Q. How were the data analysed?

Word restrictions impose limitations on the detail that can be given in any journal paper, but there should be evidence of a considered approach to data analysis.

Q. Has a computer package been used to analyse the data?

This in itself does not ensure rigour in the analysis process. It is possible to demonstrate rigour in data analysis without the use of computer packages.

Q. Is there justification as to how much data had been collected?
The researchers should seek to justify how many interviews or focus groups or other forms of qualitative data they collected.

Q. Was data saturation achieved?
Data saturation means that at the end of the analysis period, the continuing data analysis does not identify additional new themes from the data, but instead the data that is analysed merely adds to the existing themes that have emerged from previous data analysis.

Example of critical appraisal tools for qualitative studies

There are a variety of critical appraisal tools available and an internet search will enable you to view many of those accessible. As outlined above, because of the complexity of the topic, there is no one tool that is best for all qualitative research, however one of the commonly used appraisal tools is the CASP qualitative critical appraisal tool available at http://www.phru.nhs.uk/Pages/PHD/resources.htm.

Other useful resources for students are the guide to critiquing qualitative studies found in the research methods textbook by Polit and Beck (2005) and the paper by Greenhalgh and Taylor (1997) entitled *Papers that go beyond numbers (qualitative research)* which can be accessed at http://www.bmj.com/cgi/content/full/315/7110/740.

They offer the following questions:

1 Did the paper describe an important clinical problem addressed via a clearly formulated question?
2 Was a qualitative approach appropriate?
3 How were the setting and the subjects selected?
4 What was the researcher's perspective, and has this been taken into account?
5 What methods did the researcher use for collecting data – and are these described in enough detail?
6 What methods did the researcher use to analyse the data – and what quality control measures were implemented?
7 Are the results credible, and if so, are they clinically important?
8 What conclusions were drawn, and are they justified by the results?
9 Are the findings of the study transferable to other clinical settings?

Overall, for those critiquing qualitative literature, you should remember that critical appraisal of qualitative research papers is complex. Novice researchers are expected to be aware of the complexities and many different approaches to undertaking qualitative studies. Those reviewing qualitative research should become familiar with the particular approaches to qualitative study that have been used in the papers they have identified. You should then assess the rigour of the papers with the aid of a critical appraisal tool.

Key questions to ask of professional and clinical guidance and policy

As with any publication, professional and clinical guidance and policy vary in quality and should be appraised. As we have already stated, ideally, these guidelines and policy documents should be based on the best available evidence. However, it is still up to you to ensure that the advice given in the protocol is up to date and useful. In fact this should be the first question you ask of the guidelines or policy. Make a decision that from now on, you will ask yourself questions about the validity of the guidelines or policies you have to work with, rather than just accepting this at face value.

The Agree Collaboration offers guidance for the development of clinical guidelines and also a **critical appraisal tool for assessing the quality of guidelines and policy**. This is available at http://www.agreecollaboration.org/.

Hayward *et al.* (2001) have produced a document entitled **How to use a clinical practice guideline** available at http://www.cche.net/usersguides/guideline.asp which although it is more medically focussed it offers questions to ask of guidelines and policy documents. A similar tool **Practice guidelines appraisal guide** is also available at http://www.ebm.med.ualberta.ca/CPG.html. Both these guides draw upon the users guides' to evidence based medicine (see Appendix: Useful websites).

 Find out where professional and clinical guidelines specifically relevant to your practice might be published.

Key questions to ask of discussion or opinion articles (anecdotal evidence)
When you come across non-research based evidence it is important that you can recognise this and be equipped to assess its usefulness.

Q. How good is the quality of the information provided?
Do they refer to other recent sources critically?
Do they relate to their own expertise or experience?

One approach to reviewing a paper in which arguments are presented is to assess the quality of the arguments presented. This approach was originally advocated by Thouless and Thouless (1953) who discuss the use of logic in the constructed argument presented in a discussion paper. They articulate 38 'dishonest tricks' commonly used in an argument or written discussion, for example:

- Using emotionally charged words
- Making conclusive statements using words such as 'all' when 'some' would be more appropriate or 'never' when 'rarely' would be more appropriate
- Using selected instances or examples
- Misrepresentation of opposing arguments
- Not mentioning counter-arguments.

Q. Does the evidence on which the arguments are founded bear scrutiny?
If the arguments are well constructed and defensible then greater weight can be given to these arguments over those that are less well prepared and constructed. You should question the use of language, the acknowledgement of alternative approaches or lines of argument, forced analogy and false credentials.

It is important to remember that the expert opinion of a well-known figure in the area might be found to contradict established findings from empirical research. Access this report and consider George Monbiot's response to David Bellamy in the *Guardian* newspaper (2005) regarding the evidence behind the environmental threat presented by global warming:
http://www.guardian.co.uk/environment/2005/may/10/environment.columnists

George Monbiot refers to recent research findings to reinforce his argument while David Bellamy argues from his opinion only. If you applied Thouless and Thouless's (1953) criteria to these arguments, which one would have greater credibility?

Q. Who is the intended target audience?
Is it pitched appropriately?
Does it explain/define key concepts?

Example of critical appraisal tools for non-research papers (discussion and opinion papers)

Hek *et al.* (2000) report the following criteria for critiquing non-research articles:

- Is the subject relevant to the review question?
- Is it accurate?
- Is it well written and credible?

- Is it peer-reviewed in any way?
- Does it ring true?
- In what quality of journal is the report published?

Also refer to the Cottrell (2005) critical thinking checklist referred to previously.

Try and think about three things you will now do differently when reading professional literature.

Key questions to ask about information contained on websites

Q. Should I believe all information contained on websites?
The answer is of course NO! There can be no doubt that the internet contains a wealth of information that may be useful for health and social care professionals. However, as we have seen, there is also a wealth or poor quality and misleading information. It has to be acknowledged that websites are unregulated and it is possible for anybody to publish anything on an internet site. You are therefore recommended to be critical of any websites you encounter.

- The web contains many hundreds of millions of pages, including everything from rigorous research to trivia and misinformation.
- Before making use of information found on the web in your academic work, you need to make sure it is high-quality.
- You should also remember that if you use information from the web in your academic work, just like printed sources those web pages must be cited in your references of any academic work or publications (see if your organisation or university has a guide to referencing).

If you are happy with the answers you get to these questions, any material you encounter on a website can be subjected to the critical appraisal strategies as advocated by Hek *et al.* (2000), Thouless and Thouless (1953) and Cottrell (2005).

Examples of critical appraisal tools for evaluating websites

When evaluating the quality of web resources, you could also consider the following **ABC** – adapted from Howe (2001) – Accuracy, Authority, Bias, Breadth and depth, Comparison, Currency.

Accuracy – finding 'facts' or figures quoted on the web is not automatically a guarantee that the information is accurate. Can you check the information against other sources? Does it fit with what you already know? Do the authors of the page tell you where they got the information from?

Authority – who is providing the information, and what evidence do you have that they know what they are talking about?

It is not always easy to see immediately where a particular web page comes from, and an impressive-looking, whizzy web page is not necessarily a guarantee of good quality information! If you have found the page via a link or a search engine, look for a 'Home', 'Front Page', or similar icon, and follow it to try to see whether the page authors are well-known experts, and whether they provide a mission statement, 'real-world' postal address and phone number, or a bibliography of their other articles, reports or books.

Bias – As with any source of information, it is possible for a web page to appear objective, but in fact be promoting a particular standpoint. Be critical; for example, if you have found information on a particular drug, are the writers of this web page from the company which makes the drug? From a campaign group trying to get the drug banned? Or from an independent research institute?

Breadth and depth of information – How detailed is the information? What evidence is given to support it? Does it cover all relevant areas of the subject? Does the web page link to further relevant sources of information?

Currency – It is easy to assume that information on the web must be very current (up-to-date), but in fact there are now many pages on the web which have not been updated for years. How current does your information need to be? Does the page say when it was last updated? (If not, try checking the Properties or Page Info option in your Web browser and see if a date is given.) Do all the links to other sites still work? Remember, even if the page has been updated recently, all the information may not have been checked.

Comparison with other sources – To help you have confidence in the information you find, compare it with other sources of information on the subject: published statistics, journal articles, textbooks or other websites.

Fink (2005) suggests that you should ask the following questions of any websites you encounter:

- Who supports the site?
- When was it last updated?
- What authority do the authors of the site have?

There is a useful guide to evaluating web sources available at: http://www.brookes.ac.uk/library/guides/evalweb2008.pdf

There is a cartoon based checklist called QUICK (quality information check-list available at http://www.avon.k12.ct.us/enrichment/Enrich/quickgr4–0. htm which details the following questions to ask of websites:

- Is it clear who has written the information?
- Are the aims of the site clear?
- Does the site achieve its aims?
- Is the site relevant to me?
- Can the information be checked?
- When was the site produced?
- Is the information biased in any way?
- Does the site tell you about choices open to you?

Also, remember that there are a range of pre-evaluated 'subject gateways' available on the web, where experts have searched the web for high-quality, reliable information. Ask your university or workplace librarian for ideas, or try one of these gateways to get you started.

In this chapter we have considered ways of making sense of research and non-research evidence you may encounter. Overall, the purpose of critical appraisal is to enable you to make sense of the evidence you come across. It takes you from a position of '*do not believe everything you read*' to the position in which you have the skills to assess and evaluate what you read so that you can determine the strengths and weaknesses of the evidence you encounter. It is important to remember that you need to critically appraise – make sense of – all the evidence you read, whether you are using that evidence in your prac-tice or in your academic writing. However when you are using evidence in your academic work, it is useful to be mindful of the following points.

Incorporating critical appraisal into your academic writing or when debating use of evidence in practice

- Make sure that it is clear that you have read and understood the relevance and the quality of evidence you are using.
- Remember to give information about the type of evidence you are using. If it is a research study, say so, if it is a discussion article, state this.
- Resist the temptation to paraphrase or quote without evaluative comment. Make sure you give the context of the evidence you use.
- **We suggest that you don't write**: '*Jones (2009) argues that university students prefer lectures to tutorials*' (we do not know how Jones has reached this conclusion).
- **We suggest that you write instead**: '*in a questionnaire study, Jones (2009) found that 70% of students preferred lectures to tutorials*'.

- **Or instead write**: *'Jones (2009) argues that from his own experience as a student in London, there was strong feeling among his peer group that lectures were preferable to tutorials'.*

As a general rule, avoid writing a statement and then citing the author (for example Jones 2006) as the reader is completely unaware of the context of Jones work – was it a research study, based on evidence and if so which evidence or was it merely Jones' opinion. This is relevant whether you are debating the use of evidence in practice or in academic writing.

After reading this example can you identify how your writing in the past may not have fully explained the relevance and quality of the source you were using?

In summary

Once you have found your evidence, it is vital that you are able to look at it objectively and work out whether it is any good for answering your question or not. The purpose of critical appraisal is to determine the relevance, strengths and limitations of the information collected so that you can determine how helpful the evidence is in answering your question. A study might be well carried out but not very relevant to your research question. Alternatively, a study might be very relevant to your research question but not well designed or implemented. Furthermore, discussion and expert opinion might add interesting insight to your argument, but the quality of this information also needs to be assessed.

Key points

1 Remember that no research paper is perfect!
2 You need to read and re-read your papers before you can begin to critically appraise.
3 Critical appraisal is a necessary process in determining the relevance and quality of the published information related to your research question.
4 You need to distinguish between papers that report empirical findings and those that present discussion or expert opinion only.
5 You are advised to use one of the many critical appraisal tools that are available to structure your critical appraisal.

7

How to use and implement evidence in your practice and learning

What are the problems implementing the evidence into practice?
• Finding solutions to the problems of implementing evidence based practice • Evaluating the impact of evidence based changes to practice • Future visions for evidence based practice • In summary • Key points

In this chapter we will:

- Identify the problems in implementing research and other evidence into practice
- Find solutions to the difficulties you may encounter and explore the ways in which you can implement evidence in your practice setting and in your learning
- Examine strategies that can be employed when encountering an absence of evidence based practice/culture in the workplace
- Learn how to challenge and question the practice of others tactfully and constructively and deal with resistance to using evidence in practice
- Explore future visions for implementing evidence based practice.

In Chapters 1 and 2 we highlighted reasons why we need evidence based practice, including the need to provide the best possible care, issues surrounding clinical governance and the legal, professional and ethical reasons. In a society with well-informed or 'expert patients' and free and easy access to literature we are more likely to be challenged and called to account for our practice decisions.

We have then outlined the steps you need to take when you define an area for exploration, and start to search for and evaluate the evidence you find. In a way, that was the easy bit. It was certainly the logical part. It is easy to see the relevance of evidence based practice, and we would probably all prefer to be cared for by a practitioner who is up to date and accountable rather than a practitioner who is reliant on unreliable sources. Even searching for and evaluating the evidence is fairly straightforward once you have worked out how to do it.

The harder part of evidence based practice is **putting this evidence into practice.**

The Centre for Reviews and Dissemination (CRD 2008 p.90) has produced substantial guidance for professionals undertaking systematic reviews and they summarise their section on **dissemination** with the following points:

- Simply making research available does not ensure that those who need to know about it get to know about it, or can make sense of the findings.
- Dissemination is a planned and active process that can aid the transfer of research into practice.
- Dissemination should not be viewed as an adjunct but rather as an integral part of the review process and should be considered from the outset.
- CRD employs a topic-driven approach that involves targeting the right people with understandable and relevant messages, communicating via appropriate (often multiple) channels, whilst taking account of the environment in which the message will be received.

There is considerable discussion regarding what the problems might be in getting evidence into practice and as it has not currently been widely adopted by all our professions, there are clearly some practicalities that need addressing.

If you consider the list below you will see that it is the last two points we will be considering in this chapter:

Model of evidence based practice (Newman *et al.* 2006)

1 Formulate answerable question.
2 Find evidence from research.
3 Appraise for validity and usefulness.
4 Implement change.
5 Evaluate performance.

Whilst an individual professional can initiate the first three steps in their approach to evidence based practice, the process of implementation is a team effort and therefore largely dependent on the team and the culture that exists within the organisation (steps 4 and 5). Over recent years there has been a large body of literature that identifies the problems of implementation (Brown *et al.* 2008; Gerrish *et al.* 2008; Upton and Upton 2006a; Ciliska 2006; Thompson *et al.* 2004; Newman *et al.* 2000; DiCenso *et al.* 1998). There is also wide debate in the literature as to whether or not evidence based practice makes a real difference to outcomes and so we will discuss the importance of evaluating our use of evidence based practice (step 5).

As well as highlighting potential problems in implementing evidence based practice we believe that it is important to identify solutions so that the users of our services (clients, patients and their families) get the best available care.

Ask three of your peers the following question: **what is the biggest influence on the way you practise?**

Answers you obtain may include:

- Imitating role models
- Asking colleagues, peers or experts
- Going on courses/conferences
- Using the internet
- Accessing professional/clinical guidelines
- Using professional body information or standards
- Having students ask questions or challenging my practice
- Using experience rather than evidence
- Results of audits/reviews or feedback.

Think about what your own experience is of evidence based practice. Is it used to its full potential? If not, why do you think that might be?

What are the problems implementing the evidence into practice?

There are many reasons highlighted as to why evidence based practice fails to be adopted by practitioners. In this chapter we will consider some of the main reasons that are often given as to why evidence based practice is not implemented and we will look at solutions that can promote the use of an evidence based approach in our practice. In particular we will look at the following:

Lack of time/competing/higher priorities:

- Work priorities: meeting targets or deadlines, busyness, low staffing levels or skill mix.
- Family commitments, life commitments, busy lives.

Skill:

- Finding and appraising literature.
- Research is too complex to understand (jargon, language, statistics or presentation).

Access:

- Lack of access to a library or a computer.
- Too much information is available.
- Poor quality information is available.

Leadership/organisational culture/implementing change:

- Leaders have other priorities.
- There is a culture of getting the job done in some workplaces and not time for accessing and using research.
- There is no clear direction or strategic approach.
- Knowledge of evidence based practice doesn't result in changed behaviour.

Role modelling:

- Individuals may role model poor or out-of-date practice.
- Students are influenced more by practice educators more than evidence.
- Challenging the practice of others is difficult.
- Ritualistic practice is alive and well.

Relevance:

- Some value information from colleagues higher
- Some professional problems are too complex to be answered by research.
- Research doesn't take into account a holistic or individualised approach to care. 'Cook-book' approach doesn't work, too much variation in our patients.
- Research is just an excuse for rationing of care.

Finding solutions to the problems of implementing evidence based practice

'I don't have time to look for evidence. I'm just too busy . . .'

Being understaffed, too busy to think and not being able to get all our work done has been a constant issue in most health and social care workers' lives. Lack of time to find and implement evidence has been given as one of the top reasons hindering the implementation of evidence based practice (Brown *et al.* 2008; Gerrish *et al.* 2008; Upton and Upton 2006a; Ciliska 2006). Upton and Upton (2006a) highlight that for most professional groups lack of time and money were cited as the main issues.

Time management is widely discussed in the literature and strategies are offered to help us manage our time better. It is therefore worth thinking about strategies that enable us to incorporate use of evidence in our practice in a more time effective way.

Guides to help us prioritise sometimes offer the idea that we should consider what is **URGENT** and what is **IMPORTANT** when making priority decisions.

As outlined in Chapter 1 it is clear to see that using evidence to underpin our practice is important. Try considering the following:

- Consider the time that will be saved if there is a clear and consistent approach to care that will result in the best outcomes for your patient/ clients.
- Do what you can as **part of your role/daily work** rather than as an add-on.
- Be prepared for when there are slacker periods to 'find/read evidence'.

Glasziou (2009) describes an early morning informal journal club where practitioners were motivated to change practice:

- Keep articles, guidelines and other evidence available and ready to read when you have some spare time.
- Develop a questioning culture so you can share information with colleagues.
- Agree that you will ask each other why you approach a task or intervention in a particular way and try and find out if there is any evidence for that approach.
- Ask any students you have on placement to talk about what they are learning in university (ask them to bring in relevant articles/lecture notes or even do a presentation to the team).
- See if your student has time/need to investigate a clinical issue and see if they would be interested in doing a literature review on a topic relevant to your practice.

Stone and Rowles (2007) describe how a student research utilisation project was used to increase staff awareness of research findings and save staff time. Consider the following suggestions:

- Ask experts/specialists for any summaries/guidelines they know of relating to your speciality (remember to critically appraise them).
- Start by accessing sites that contain systematic reviews or clinical knowledge summaries or evidence based practice journals rather than individual articles or books.

Haynes (2007) offers a staged approach to finding evidence and suggests that we search at the highest possible level (decision support systems or systematic reviews) before looking any further. They therefore support arguments made earlier in this book that reviews of research are a particularly useful resource. Consider the following suggestions:

- Take turns in finding out the best available evidence on a topic and present it at team meetings.
- Ensure any staff member who attends a study day/conference or course feeds back to the wider team any implications for practice.
- Try and build in the evidence base for your other priorities (targets, projects or strategies) and see how it relates to improving patient/client outcomes.
- Consider if attending a clinical conference or doing a course would be a faster/more effective way of ensuring your practice is up to date.

Regarding home life and family commitments it is worth ensuring you adopt good time management skills in your home life too. Planning so that you can achieve a healthy work–life balance is important so that you can prioritise and enjoy important social and family events. However, being a professional does mean keeping up to date and so you may also want to consider how you can plan in time for your own professional development. It is often difficult to study or concentrate at home so consider:

- Coming in a little early for your work and accessing a workplace library.
- Staying at work for a little later to read an article or access evidence for your practice.
- Building in time for your development once a month.
- Setting goals to motivate you such as journal clubs or projects that involve working with others.
- Setting aside a time/place at home for you to update yourself.
- Explain to those close to you why you need to have time to develop yourself.

'I'm just not any good at finding evidence. I don't know where to start!'
Hopefully, after reading this book, you will feel equipped to search for evidence.

Upton and Upton (2006a) carried out a survey of the knowledge and use of evidence based practice by 14 allied health professionals in the United Kingdom, and Hadley *et al.* (2008) incorporated complementary and alternative health care professionals in their survey. In these studies, they found similarities and differences between professional groups and some of these can be attributed to the varying approaches to education and policy and also the amount of evidence available.

> **Example skills** such as formulating a PICOT question, using databases and information technology, combining and saving searches, understanding research methods, recognising relevance of hierarchies of evidence for different questions, using appraisal tools, reading research (understanding the language) and interpreting statistics.

Lack of skill is likely to act as a barrier to accessing and implementing evidence in our practice.

There are many professionals whose initial training did not incorporate using information technology to search for evidence. Many individuals say that they have never studied research methods or were not taught how to adopt a critical approach to literature (this sometimes depends on where or when we trained). Most health and social care professionals are now educated to a minimum of diploma level and how evidence based practice is incorporated into curricula will vary. Ciliska (2006) identifies many of the issues relating to implementing evidence based practice and questions if all practitioners need the skills for evidence based practice or if specialists should take on the role. We argue that it is vital for all practitioners to develop the minimum skills and an awareness to implement an evidence based approach. Whilst ideally guidelines and policy are evidence based, there will always be a large area of professional practice which is not governed by policy or guidelines and it is here that practitioners should draw on their own skills of implementing an evidence based approach.

Dawes *et al.* (2005 p.3) in their consensus statement agree that:

it is a minimum requirement that all practitioners understand the principles of EBP, implement evidence-based policies, and have a critical attitude to their own practice and to evidence. Without these skills and attitudes, health care professionals will find it difficult to provide best practice. Teachers, commissioners, and those in positions of leadership will require appraisal skills that come with higher training and continued use.

Part of being accountable for our practice is to recognise and address any limitations in our knowledge and skills and seek out further education.

As discussed in Chapter 2, the amount of information available for us to access is now considerable. Upton and Upton (2006b) offer an evidence based practice questionnaire which, although aimed at nurses, would be relevant to other professionals. It aims to measure self-report of knowledge, practice and attitudes to evidence based practice. They conclude that there is a clear and logical link between the attitudes, knowledge and actual practice of evidence based practice and that the tool can be used to measure the implementation of evidence based practice. In order to generate excitement and to address the specific area of lack of skill in formulating research questions, Brown et al. (2008) organised a competition in their organisation for asking clinical questions as this was an area highlighted where staff lacked skill.

Complete the questionnaire offered by Upton and Upton (2006b) to help you self assess what may be influencing your use of evidence based practice. Also consider what Dawes et al. (2005) highlight as the minimum standard educational requirements.

- Don't wait until you need the skills (for a course or a project) before you learn them. There will be greater pressure on you then.
- If you are a student, access the library tutorials when they are offered.
- Practise searching for evidence when you write an academic assignment rather than relying on the reference list.
- Discuss with your peers how confident they are in their knowledge of practice (it is likely that most will feel the same as you).
- Read research and/or research books so that you become more familiar with the language and terminology used. Use a glossary or thesaurus where available.
- Discuss at your appraisal any professional development needs you have in relation to searching/appraising information and ensure your manager knows where you lack knowledge for your practice.
- Find out if your organisation offers any training on evidence based practice.
- Ask your manager if you can go on library training sessions or have study time to do online tutorials where available.
- See if there is a team member or student on placement who has more skill in searching and appraising than you and see if they can help you develop these skills.
- Have a go! Use widely available sites such as www.cochrane.org and http://www.library.nhs.uk and just play around to see what is available.

If you are involved in education, you can promote an evidence based approach in the following ways:

- Ensure that the skills for evidence based practice are clear in the learning outcomes of the courses.
- Introduce evidence based practice early on in the curriculum.
- Offer regular, timetabled library skills sessions.
- Ensure that clinical skills sessions have a clear rationale and relevant research is available for students.
- Invite practitioners to contribute (as facilitators or patients) in the simulated learning environment.
- Ensure that evidence based practice is related explicitly to clinical decision making to ensure that students are more likely to engage with it.
- Make the use of evidence and critical appraisal evident in the grading criteria and in both academic and practice based assignments (competencies).
- Encourage students to use subject librarians and study skills support available at the university.
- Ensure that role modelling and evidence based practice are discussed as part of practice educator update days.
- Encourage lecturers to make explicit how the research that underpins teaching is appraised (and so they role model critical appraisal in their teaching).

The important point is that a promoting an evidence based approach requires commitment and implementation from everyone involved – from students, mentors and lecturers to those writing the guidelines and making policy decisions.

Richardson and Dowding (2005) provide seven suggestions as to how teachers can develop their skills in this area:

1 Refining their own skills in evidence based practice
2 Improving access to resources
3 Anticipating recurrent questions and find evidence in advance
4 Keeping concise summaries of the evidence
5 Assembling decision aids for more complex decisions
6 Keep some 'how to' guides readily available
7 Developing 'teaching awareness through reflection' to help recognise the teaching moments.

'We don't have access to computers at work so it's difficult to access evidence'

In Chapter 5 we explain how to find your evidence. However it is clear that access to up-to-date evidence is a problem for busy practitioners.

We have discussed earlier how developing confidence and competence in the skills in searching for and reading research will clearly help with this accessibility. If you are familiar with the databases and know how to search, it will be easier for you to access evidence. If organisations can help practitioners to access information then this is more effective than practitioners working alone. For example, are there computers in your workplace and are staff encouraged to use the internet to access evidence during work time? Perry and Mclaren (2003) describe a multi-professional project where the implementation of evidence relating to nutrition in acute stroke was targeted. They found that despite limited resources and a challenging health care climate, changes in practice can be made.

- Find out what is available from your organisation:
  - Do you have access to a computer with internet access?
  - Is priority given to students and staff to access sources of evidence in the workplace?
  - Are you encouraged to find out the evidence base for your practice?
  - Is there a library you can join?
  - Do you subscribe to any journals (hard copy or electronically)?
  - Is there a local intranet (in house computer network that only those authorised can access)?
  - If there is, does it contain policy, guidance or links to useful sites?
  - Are there any local projects going on relating to using evidence?
- Ask an experienced colleague or educationalist which journals are considered good quality and where you might be able to find them.
- If you have access to a library with electronic full-text journals consider setting up email alerts (a regular email of contents pages) so you can regularly check for relevant content.
- We also recognise that accessibility to resources makes a considerable difference and for a wide range of students, being able to access information from home is considered an important factor. Part of being able to access sources includes gaining information technology skills.

'When I do find evidence I can't understand it'

Access to evidence includes both physical access to computers or libraries and also accessibility – that is, how practitioners feel able to use the evidence in terms of its readability and understanding. If you find evidence but then cannot understand it, then the evidence is of little use to you. Iles and Davidson (2006) carried out a 'self-reporting' survey of physiotherapists' practice in relation to evidence based practice and problems with accessibility of the evidence were highlighted. Hopefully, after reading this book, you will feel more confident in understanding what you read; you will get better at this the more often you read professional literature. If you find it difficult to make sense of what you read, try showing the evidence to a colleague, another professional or a student and see if together you can make sense of it. If the evidence seems controversial in any way, you could discuss the evidence as part of a journal club or other informal meeting.

'My manager does not support me trying to use an evidence based approach'

There is currently, and has been for some time, an understanding of how **leadership** influences a professional learning environment (Gopee 2008). More recently, terms such as 'communities of practice', 'learning organisations' or 'learning communities' have been developed, which describe a more coherent approach to professional learning and development. Rycroft Malone (2008) in her editorial discusses leadership and evidence based practice and how research can provide a more robust basis for the assertion that leaders play an important role in the use of evidence in practice, be that positively or negatively.

Rycroft Malone asserts that we should:

- Invest in key individuals at multiple levels of the organisation and develop their leadership capacity and ability to support their colleagues in the development of evidence based practice
- Continue to study the influence that those in informal or formal leadership positions have on implementation efforts so that the knowledge base continues to develop.

This supports the view mentioned earlier, that the input and commitment of all staff is required if we are to foster an evidence based approach. Ciliska (2006) and Newman *et al.* (2000) identified the importance of the organisation in providing the structure to support the development of an evidence based approach. This illustrates the need to be aware of the **organisational culture** in which you are working, either as a student or as a registered professional so that you can plan your strategies to achieve evidence based practice.

Carry out a **SWOT analysis** of your workplace – what are the Strengths, Weaknesses, Opportunities and Threats in relation to implementing evidence based practice?

Parahoo (2000) found that lack of manager support was one of the main barriers to the uptake of research findings and Newman *et al.* (2000) found that a ward manager could act as a negative role model if they did not prioritise evidence based practice above their other roles. Gifford *et al.* (2007) describe the leadership activities of managers that might influence use of research evidence by their staff. From a review of 12 quantitative studies they showed that influential leadership activities included managerial support, policy revisions and auditing. Within qualitative studies, role modelling and valuing of research by leaders were found to facilitate research use.

What influences practitioners implementing change in practice has been the subject of a Cochrane systematic review (Cheater *et al.* 2005) and they concluded that due to a small number of studies, it is also not possible to determine whether strategies tailored to overcome organisational barriers are more effective than those that were not. It is also not clear whether all barriers or important barriers were identified and addressed by the strategies. More research about how to identify and overcome barriers is needed. Newman *et al.* (2000) introduced a range of systems including use of action research, role clarification for staff in a professional development role and clinical supervision with the intention to influence organisational change and found some difficulties in sustaining the positive changes which clearly relate to many of the problems identified in this chapter. As you can see, ways of promoting and enhancing an evidence based approach are yet to be fully evaluated, but we can ask the following questions for promoting a positive environment:

Consider the following:

- Does the leader of your workplace or place of study invite a questioning/ challenging approach and does that influence all staff/learners?
- Is the leadership committed to adopting an evidence based approach to practice?
- Is there an organisational or strategic approach to adopting new evidence or practice guidance, policy or protocols?
- How is change introduced into practice and who is involved in developing and evaluating the implementation of change?

As we have already identified, one of the key influences highlighted by practitioners is time. Time is our most precious resource and busy practitioners 'keep their heads down' and do what they need to do to get the job done. Evidence based practice seems to be an optional extra. This then becomes a wider organisational issue where strong leadership has potential to influence change. Managers should ensure that **staffing levels should incorporate time** for developing and implementing and evidence based approach to practice. This then shows that professional development is valued within the organisation.

Clinical and professional leaders need to argue for better staffing that includes time for continued professional development.

There are many new and emerging roles where practitioners are able to have real influence on clinical decision making such as consultant roles, specialist practitioners, specialists or leads in education and professional development. Guest *et al.* (2002) reports that such practitioners have made some inroads into developing practice. Leaders should consider how such roles may be best used within their organisations.

'I worry if I am a good enough role model for evidence based practice?'
In our experience as practitioners and lecturers the biggest influence on professional practice often comes from **role modelling** from other professionals.

Consider if your practice was observed and copied by a learner what would you be proud of and are there any aspects of your practice that you might be uncertain about?

We are aware of the importance of role modelling and the significance students place on what they learn in practice (Fowler 2008; Gopee 2008; Donaldson and Carter 2005). In fact, in our experience, when asked where they learn most of their practical skills, students constantly tell us that it is from their practice educators – rather than from textbooks, journals, university sessions or other evidence based sources.

There is one important (if obvious) point to be made: **role modelling works well if the role model is drawing on current evidence based information and research to inform their practice.** However, if we role model unsafe or out-of-date practices then ritualistic practice (as discussed in Chapter 2) thrives. If practitioners are not up to date, this is likely to have a big influence on student learning. Yet there is concern that practice educators are not adequately supported in their role and not always able to support their students (Nettleton and Bray 2008; Myall *et al.* 2008). There is the potential for practice to be based on ritual rather than evidence if both students and practitioners fail to be open to challenge in their practice.

If students on pre- or post-qualifying courses adopt the practices of those supervising them without question then we are continuing ritualistic practices which may be out of date or even dangerous.

As a learner or as a professional who is accountable for your own practice, you can see that the role of clinical judgement could lead to differing of opinion in clinical practice. One experienced practitioner might interpret a situation in one way and suggest one evidence based course of action, and another might suggest a different evidence based approach. As Rolfe (1999 p.437) points out:

An experienced practitioner is someone who has accumulated a body of experiential knowledge from many years of practice. But like anything, experiential knowledge can be used poorly or wisely and there are many practitioners with twenty years or more experience who fail to make good use of it. What separates the experienced nurse from the expert is the wise application of experiential knowledge.

More recently, Thompson (2003) highlights that, whilst it is necessary to draw on experience for our practice decisions, it is not a sufficient basis. This is why as a professional yourself or if you are in a student role, you need to **develop a rationale for your own practice** and should not act merely because you have been told to act in a certain way. This will make you a more effective role model.

Strategies you can adopt are:

- Ask colleagues or practice assessors for a rationale for their care decisions and judge the rationale they give you, check it out for yourself to see if you would make the same decision based on the evidence. If they are unable to give you a rationale, discuss how you might work on this together.
- If you supervise students then you could find out what evidence they are using in the theory part of their course (they have access to up-to-date lectures, seminars and library resources) and you may be able to learn from them.
- Think about how you and your team react to having your practice challenged. Is it seen as a way of professionally developing or as a personal criticism? Could you do more to invite challenge to your practice (give permission)?
- Encouraging your clinical area to pre-plan evidence based practice approach regarding frequently occurring situations so that responses are evidence based (Richardson and Dowding 2005).
- Volunteer to help out with teaching clinical/professional skills at your local university (this can be mutually beneficial in helping bridge the theory–practice gap).

'How do I challenge the practice of others?'
Most people would welcome feedback to improve their practice, although it is worth recognising that in a busy working environment or if practice is challenged in an untactful way then our natural reaction would be to be defensive.

Think of a time when someone has challenged you about something that was entirely justifiable. If they approached you in a tactful way you were probably more likely to accept what they were saying than if they confronted you directly.

In the Knowledge and Skills Framework (DH 2004b) under the dimension of People and Personal Development (level 4) the Department of Health identifies the need to encourage others to make realistic self-assessments of their application of knowledge and skills and in challenging complacency and actions which are not in patients' or the public's interest. It is also mentioned in the domain of Health, Safety and Security (level 3) challenging people who put themselves or others at risk.

The British Association of Social Workers (BASW 2002 p.11) in their Code of Ethics assert that social workers should:

> Familiarise themselves with the complaints and whistleblowing procedures of their workplace . . . addressing suspected or confirmed professional misconduct, incompetence, unethical behavior or negligence by a colleague through the appropriate organisational, professional or legal channels.

Consider what you would do if you spotted unsafe or out-of-date practice by a colleague, practice educator or student.

- Discuss with colleagues/practice educators/students in advance what you should do if you see practice that conflicts with evidence you are aware of.
- Consider if the practice is unsafe or inappropriate and your role as an advocate for your patients or clients; bring the evidence with you before you challenge them.
- Before you challenge the practice of others consider what evidence you have (might there be things you are unaware of, for example, context, more than one approach or different values?).
- Consider the setting; avoid challenging another professional in public unless the practice is unsafe. Ask to speak to them privately.
- Consider asking questions rather than making accusations about practice.
- Provide any evidence you have for the practice issue.
- Ask for their perspective on the issue/your observations.
- Give the person a chance to consider your view or question.

We have produced guidelines for students regarding how to manage concerns in practice placements. Available at http://shsc.brookes.ac.uk/plu/guidelines-for-managing-concerns-in-practice-placements

'Is the evidence I find really relevant?'
It is unquestionable that there has been a recent increased interest in evidence based practice indicated by the growth of evidence based organisations and centres (see Chapter 1), specific evidence based journals and access to articles online (downloads) (Ciliska 2006). Presentations at conferences also now include more clinical research (Tod *et al.* 2004).

There is evidence that how relevant practitioners see implementing an evidence based approach to their practice influences the value they place on it, and their motivations to develop skills or spend time on it. Upton and Upton (2006b) found in a postal questionnaire that practitioners generally had a positive attitude to evidence based practice although many of the problems outlined earlier in this chapter influenced their ability to use it to its full potential.

However, some practitioners may still feel that information from colleagues is quicker to access and in a fast-paced setting this may be the only way of solving practice problems and so research seems less relevant to the reality of practice. If this continues to be the case, we will not be able to cultivate an evidence based practice environment. As accountable practitioners, we should be checking out that information as soon as we can to ensure our own practice is up to date.

Practice problems are often complex and messy and so finding evidence based answers to more complex decisions can be challenging. As practitioners strive to adopt an individualised and person centred approach to care then there are those that might argue that evidence based practice tries to standardise care (a cook-book approach). This may be seen in the use of care pathways, protocols and guidance that is followed without question. However, if such tools and guidance are used flexibly alongside professional judgement and patient preferences, evidence based practice then becomes relevant and appropriate. It remains up to your own professional judgement as to whether you apply the evidence that you find, remembering that you are accountable for the practice you deliver.

As we have discussed earlier, it will also often be the case that there is not appropriate evidence to underpin your practice. When this is the case, this must be acknowledged.

Evaluating the impact of evidence based changes to practice

Evidence based practice is likely to be valued more highly if practitioners can see benefit in **patient/client outcomes**. Thomas *et al.* (2009) in a Cochrane review across professional groups conclude that the issuing of clinical guidelines may reduce variations in practice and improve patient care. They found that, despite limited research, there is some evidence that guidelines can improve care but further research is needed. If problems are solved more quickly, if interventions were more effective or if quality of life was improved then practitioners are more likely to utilise and see the relevance of using evidence for their practice. It is therefore important that changes to practice are monitored. This can be done through a variety of approaches:

- Recording of base-line or pre-change information
- Monitoring and reporting locally the impact of changes
- Use of national targets/standards
- Local or larger scale audit
- Evaluation research which can include clinical impact or cost/benefit.

Future visions for evidence based practice

There is clearly considerable work that needs to be done in order to improve the implementation of evidence into the real world of practice.

Ciliska (2006) hopes that we will successfully bridge the research transfer gap in order to make decisions related to practice, management and policy. She recognises that access to resources, and development of clear strategies for managing change and overcoming barriers are needed. She also identifies that education at all levels for staff is key, so too is the need to evaluate the effectiveness of evidence based practice. Dawes *et al.* (2005) conclude that evidence based practice requires a health care infrastructure committed to best practice, and able to provide full and rapid access to electronic databases at the point of care delivery. Tod *et al.* (2004 p.215) argue that it is a time of opportunity if practitioners 'wish to visit the world of evidence based practice they will be pushing against an open door'. They suggest that strategies are needed to make things happen such as:

- Establishing clinically focussed journal clubs
- Developing organisational evidence based practice groups
- Professionals taking the lead in developing protocols or care pathways.

Brown *et al.* (2008) found that respondents of their questionnaire had individual visions of what would facilitate research utilisation. These ideas included:

- An environment of open communication and exchange of ideas
- Effort applauded
- New ideas praised
- Emphasis on a team approach to problem solving
- Collaboration
- Research shared at staff meetings
- Updates in a newsletter
- Champions
- Research posters
- Discussion forums
- Journal clubs.

Thompson *et al.* (2005) suggest targeted implementation strategies would be the most fruitful. They suggest that strategies that relate to clinical decision making should be taken into account.

In summary

In this book we have identified that developing an evidence based practice approach is both a personal and an organisational goal. We need to develop both if we are to promote the use of evidence in our professional practice. As an individual, it is vital that you understand why evidence based practice is an important aspect of delivering high standards of practice. You need to develop and feel confident about your skills of finding and evaluating evidence. All professionals need to be aware of the need for evidence based practice and to have the skills to search for and understand the evidence they find. Then you need to be working within an organisational culture that is open and receptive to change and prepared to embrace the concept of using evidence in practice. Although the second stage is dependent on the culture of the organisation, the culture of the organisation is dependent on the individuals within it. Therefore there is much that you as an individual and together with your colleagues can do to support the development of this culture as outlined in this chapter.

We hope that you have found this introduction to evidence based practice useful and relevant to your professional lives.

Key points

1 Developing evidence based practice requires the practitioner to have the skills of finding and evaluating evidence.
2 This requires the motivation and dedication of the individual practitioner to achieve this.
3 Developing an evidence based practice approach also requires an organisational culture of accepting change.
4 Do not underestimate your individual contribution to this organisational culture as an individual – even as a student. Remember that the organisation is made up of individuals.

Glossary

Abstract: A summary of a research or discussion paper.

Action Research: A study carried out in a setting in which the results are implemented and evaluated within that setting.

Case control study: A study in which people with a specific condition (cases) are compared to people without this condition (controls) to compare the frequency of the occurrence of the exposure that might have caused the disease.

CONSORT statement: A statement that describes the information that should be included in the report of a trial.

Critical appraisal: A process by which the quality of evidence is assessed.

Critical appraisal tool: A checklist used to assess the quality of evidence.

Cohort study: A study in which two or more groups or cohorts are followed up to examine whether exposures measured at the beginning lead to outcomes, such as disease.

Confidence Interval: Confidence intervals are usually (but arbitrarily) 95% confidence intervals. A reasonable, though strictly incorrect interpretation, is that the 95% confidence interval gives the range in which the population effect lies.

Convenience sample: A sample that is obtained due to convenience factors – for example, all those attending a seminar are invited to fill in a questionnaire.

Descriptive statistics: Statistics such as means, medians, standard deviations, that describe aspects of the data, such as central tendency (mean or median) or its dispersion (standard deviation).

Discussion papers: A paper presenting an argument or discussion.

Dissertation: A document presenting the main findings from a piece of academic work.

Empirical research: Research the opposite of empirical is theoretical. Empirical research is research which is based on observation or experiment.

Essay: A short piece of academic writing on a selected topic.

Ethnography: Qualitative research approach which involves the study of culture/way of life of participants.

Evidence based practice: Practice which is based on the best available evidence, moderated by patient preferences.

Exclusion criteria: Criteria that are set in order to focus the searching strategy for a literature review (e.g. not children, not acute care episodes).

Generalise: To apply the findings of a study to another population.

Grounded theory: Qualitative research approach that involves the generation of theory.

Hierarchy of evidence: A grading system for assessing the quality of evidence.

Inclusion and exclusion criteria: Criteria that are set in order to focus the searching strategy for a literature review (e.g. research from the past 5 years, published in English).

Inferential statistics: Statistics that are used to infer findings from the sample population to the wider population, usually meaning statistical tests.

Meta-analysis: A process by which quantitative data with similar properties is combined to produce a weighted average of all the results.

Meta-ethnography: A process by which qualitative data is combined.

Meta-study: A process by which qualitative data is combined.

Narrative review: A literature review that is not undertaken according to a predefined and systematic approach.

Non-empirical evidence: Evidence that is not based on the findings of research.

Phenomenology: Qualitative research approach in which the participants 'lived experience' is explored.

Purposive sampling: Sampling strategy used by qualitative researchers who are looking for a sample that is 'fit for the purposes' of the study in question.

P values: p for probability. The p value is the probability of observing results or results more extreme than those observed if the null hypothesis was true.

Qualitative research: Research that involves an in-depth understanding of the reasons for and meanings of human behaviour.

Quantitative research: Research that involves counting.

Random sampling: A sampling strategy in which everyone in a given population has an equal chance of being selected and that probability is independent of any other person selected.

Randomisation: The process of allocating individuals randomly to groups in a trial.

Randomised controlled trial: A trial which has randomly assigned groups in order to determine the effectiveness of an intervention(s) which is given to one/ two of the groups.

Research question: A question set by researchers at the outset of a study, to be addressed in the study.

Research methodology: The process undertaken in order to address the research question.

Secondary sources: A source which is not derived from an eyewitness account of a situation.

Snowball sampling: A sampling strategy in which who/what is involved in the study (sample) is determined according to the needs of the study as the investigation progresses.

Stratification: Stratification is when the sample is divided into groups that have the same value, for example, stratifying by age means putting people of the same age or age group together.

Systematic review: A review of the literature that is undertaken according to a defined and systematic approach.

Theoretical sampling: An approach to sampling in grounded theory where the sampling strategy evolves as the study progresses, according to the needs of the study and the developing theory.

References

Aveyard H (2004) The patient who refuses nursing care, *Journal of Medical Ethics* 30: 346–50

Aveyard H (2007) *Doing a Literature Review in Health and Social Care*. Open University Press: Maidenhead

Barbour RS (2001) Checklists for improving rigour in qualitative research. A case of the tail wagging the dog? *British Medical Journal* 322: 1115–17

Benner, P. (1984) *From Novice To Expert*. Addison Wesley Publishing Company: New York

Benner P and Tanner CA (1987) Clinical judgement: How expert nurses use intuition, *American Journal of Nursing* 87(1): 23–31

Boynton PM and Greenhalgh T (2004) Hands-on guide to questionnaire research; selecting, designing, and developing your questionnaire, *British Medical Journal* 328: 1312–15

British Association of Social Workers (2002) Code of Ethics. BASW: London

Brown CE, Wickline MA, Ecoff L and Galser D (2008) Nursing practice, knowledge, attitudes and perceived barriers to evidence based practice at an academic medical centre, *Journal of Advanced Nursing* 65(2): 371–81

Burls A (2009) *What is critical appraisal?* (2nd edn) Haywood Medical Communications: Newmarket UK

Centre for Reviews and Dissemination (2008) *Systematic Reviews: Guidance for Undertaking Reviews in Health Care*. CRD: York

Cheater F, Baker R, Gillies C *et al.* (2005) Tailored interventions to overcome identified barriers to change: effects on professional practice and health care outcomes, *Cochrane Database of Systematic Reviews* 2005, Issue 3: CD005470. DOI: 10.1002/14651858.CD005470.http://www.cochrane.org/reviews/en/ab005470.html

Ciliska D (2006) Evidence based nursing: how far have we come? What's next? *Evidence-based Nursing* 9: 38–40

Cottrell S (2005) *Critical Thinking Skills*. Palgrave MacMillan: Basingstoke

Crombie I (2006) *Pocket Guide to Critical Appraisal*. BMJ Publishing Group: London

Dawes M, Summerskill W, Glasziou P *et al.* (2005) Sicily statement on evidence-based practice, *BMC Medical Education* 5(1): 1–7

Demicheli V, Jefferson T, Rivetti A and Price D (2006) Vaccines for measles, mumps and rubella in children, *Cochrane Database of Systematic Reviews* Issue 2. The Cochrane Collaboration. Chichester: John Wiley and Sons

Department of Health (1998) *A First Class Service*. DH. London

Department of Health (2004a) *Patient and public involvement in health*. DH: London

Department of Health (2004b) *Knowledge and skills framework and the development review process*. DH: London

DiCenso A, Cullum N and Ciliska D (1998) Implementing evidence-based nursing: some misconceptions, *Evidence-Based Nursing* 1: 38–9

Diggle L and Deeks J (2006) Effect of needle size on immunogenicity and reactogenicity of vaccines in infants: randomized controlled trial, *British Medical Journal* 333: 571

Dimond B (2008) *Legal Aspects of Nursing*. Longman: Harlow

Doll R and Hill AB (1954) The mortality of doctors in relation to their smoking habits, *British Medical Journal* 228: 1451–5

Donaldson JH and Carter D; (2005) The value of role modelling: perceptions of undergraduate and diploma nursing (adult) students. *Nurse Education in Practice*, Nov; 5 (6): 353–9

Easterbrook PJ, Berlin JA, Gopalan R and Matthews DR (1991) Publication bias in clinical trials, *Lancet* 337(8746): 867–72

Eckmanns T, Bessert J, Behnke M, Gastmeier P and Ruden H (2006) Compliance with antiseptic hand rub use in intensive care units: the Hawthorne effect, *Infection Control and Hospital Epidemiology* 27(9): 931–4

Elliott N (2003) Portfolio creation, action research and the learning environment: a study from probation, *Qualitative Social Work* 2(3): 327–45

Ellis J, Mulligan I, Rowe J and Sackett DL (1995) Inpatient general medicine is evidence based, *Lancet* 346(8972): 407–10

Fineout-Overholt E and Johnston L (2005) Teaching EBP: Asking searchable, answerable clinical questions, *World Views on Evidence-based Nursing* 2(3): 157–60

Fink A (2005) *Conducting Research Literature Reviews*. Sage Publications: Thousand Oaks

Fleming ND and Mills C (1992) Not another inventory, rather a catalyst for reflection, *To Improve the Academy* 11: 137

Fowler D (2008) Student midwives and accountability. Are midwives good role models? *British Journal of Midwifery* 16(2): 100–4

Gerrish K, Ashworth P, Lacey A and Bailey J (2008) Developing evidence-based practice: experiences of senior and junior clinical nurses. *Journal of Advanced Nursing* 62(1): 62–73

Gill P, Dowell AC, Neal RD, Smith N and Heywood P (1996) Evidence based general practice: a retrospective study of interventions in one general training practice, *British Medical Journal* 312: 819–21

Girou E, Loyeau S, Legrand P, Oppein F and Brun-Buisson C (2002) Efficacy of handrubbing with alcohol based solution versus standard handwashing with antiseptic soap: randomised clinical trial, *British Medical Journal* 325: 362

Glasziou P (2009) Applying evidence – what is the next action? *Evidence-based nursing* 12: 7–8

Goldacre B (2008) *Bad Science*. HarperCollins: London

Gopee N (2008) *Mentoring and Supervision in Healthcare*. Sage Publications: London

Greenhalgh T (1997a) How to read a paper. Papers that summarise other papers, *British Medical Journal* 315: 672–5

Greenhalgh T (1997b) How to read a paper. Statistics for the non statistician, *British Medical Journal* 315: 422–5

Greenhalgh T and Peacock R (2005) Effectiveness and efficiency of search methods in systematic reviews of complex evidence. audit of primary sources, *British Medical Journal* 331: 1064–5

Greenhalgh T and Taylor R (1997) How to read a paper. Papers that go beyond numbers (qualitative research), *British Medical Journal* 315: 740–3

Guardian (2005) Comment. Tuesday 10 May

Guest C, Smith L, Bradshaw M, Hardcastle W (2002) Facilitating interprofessional learning for medical and nursing students in clinical practice, *Learning in Health and Social Care* 1(3): 132–8

Hadley J, Hassan J and Khan KS (2008) Knowledge and beliefs concerning evidence-based practice amongst complementary and alternative medicine health care practitioners and allied health care professionals: A questionnaire survey, *BMC Complementary and Alternative Medicine* 8(45) http://www.biomedcentral.com/1472–6882/8/45

Hawker S, Payne S, Kerr C, Hardey M and Powell J (2002) Appraising the evidence. Reviewing disparate data systematically, *Qualitative Health Research* 12(9): 1284–99

Haynes B (2007) Of studies, synthesis, synopsis, summaries and systems: the '5S' evolution of information services for evidence based health care decisions, *Evidence-based Nursing* 10: 6–7

Hayward RSA, Wilson MC, Tunis SR, Bass EB and Guyatt G (2001) How to use a clinical practice guideline. Available at http://www.cche.net/usersguides/guideline.asp (accessed 14 March 2009)

Health Professions Council (HPC) (2008) *Standards of Conduct, Performance and Ethics.* Available at http://www.hpc-uk.org/aboutregistration/standards/

Hek G, Langton H and Blunden G (2000) Systematically searching and reviewing literature, *Nurse Researcher* 7(3): Spring

Howe W (2001) Evaluating quality. Available at http://www.walthowe.com/navnet/quality.html (accessed 14 March 2009)

Iles R and Davidson (2006) Evidence based practice: a survey of physiotherapists' current practice, *Physiotherapy Research International* 11(2): 93–103

Kirschning S, von Kardorff E and Merai K (2007) Internet use by the families of cancer patients – help for disease management? *Journal of Public Health* 15(1): 23–8

Knipschild P (1994) Systematic reviews: some examples, *British Medical Journal* 309: 719–21

Lincoln YS and Guba EG (1985) *Naturalistic Inquiry.* Sage Publications: Beverly Hills, CA

Lloyd-Jones M (2004) Application of systematic review methods to qualitative research: practical issues, *Journal of Advanced Nursing* 48(3): 271–8

Moher D, Schulz KF and Altman DG (2001) The CONSORT statement. Revised recommendations for improving the quality of reports of parallel groups randomised trials, *Annals of Internal Medicine* 134(8): 657–62

Mulrow CD, Cook DJ and Davidoff F (1997) Systematic reviews. Critical links in the great chain of evidence. *Annals of Internal Medicine* 126(5): 389–91

Myall M, Levett-Jones T and Lathlean J (2008) Mentorship in contemporary practice: the experiences of nursing students and practice mentors, *Journal of Clinical Nursing* 17(14): 1834–42

Nettleton P and Bray L (2008) Current mentorship schemes might be doing our students a disservice, *Nurse Education in Practice* 8(3): 205–12

Newman M, Papadopoulos I and Melifonwu R (2000) Developing organisational systems and culture to support evidence based practice: the experience of the evidence based practice ward. *Evidence-based Nursing* 3: 103–4

Newman M, Thompson C and Roberts AP (2006) Helping practitioners understand the contribution of qualitative research to evidence based practice. *Evidence-based Nursing* 9: 4–7

Nursing and Midwifery Council (NMC) (2008) *Standards of Conduct, Performance and Ethics.* Available at http://www.nmc-uk.org/aSection.aspx?SectionID=45

Oldershaw M (2009) *What are adult nursing students' attitudes towards patients with HIV/*

AIDS and what can be done to improve attitudes? Unpublished BSc (hons) dissertation, School of Health and Social Care, Oxford Brookes University

Parahoo K (2000) Barriers to, and facilitations of research utilisation among nurses in Northern Ireland, *Journal of Advanced Nursing* 9: 38–40

Parsons AC, Shraim M, Inglis J, Aveyard P and Hajek P (2008) Interventions for preventing weight gain after smoking cessation, *Cochrane Database of Systematic Reviews* 2009, Issue 1: CD006219. DOI: 10.1002/14651858.CD006219.pub2

Pauling L (1986) *How to Live Longer and Feel Better.* Oregon State University Press: Oregon

Perry L and McLaren S (2003) Implementing evidence based guidelines for nutrition support in acute stroke, *Evidence-based Nursing* 6: 68–71

Philpin FM (2002) Rituals in nursing – a critical commentary, *Journal of Advanced Nursing* 38(2): 144–51

Polit DF and Beck C (2005) *Essentials of Nursing Research.* Lippincott Williams & Wilkins: New York

Popay J, Rogers A and Williams G (1998) Rationale and standards for the systematic review of qualitative literature in health services research, *Qualitative Health Research* 8(3): 341–51

Richardson WS and Dowding RN (2005) Teaching evidence based practice on foot, *Evidence-based Nursing* 8: 100–3

Rochon PA, Gurwitz JH, Sykora K *et al.* (2005) Reader's guide to critical appraisal of cohort studies. 1. Role and design, *British Medical Journal* 330: 895–7

Rolfe G (1999) Insufficient evidence: the problems of evidence-based medicine, *Nurse Education Today* 19: 422–42

Russell CK and Gregory DM (2003) Evaluation of qualitative research studies, *Evidence-based Nursing* 6: 36–40

Rycroft Malone J (2008) Leadership and the use of evidence in practice, *World Views on Evidence-based Nursing* 5(1): 1–2

Sackett DL, Rosenberg WMC, Muir Gray JA, Haynes RB and Richardson WS (1996) Evidence based medicine. What it is and what it isn't, *British Medical Journal* 312: 71–2

Sandelowski M and Barroso J (2002) Reading qualitative studies, *International Journal of Qualitative Studies* 1: 1

Smith R (1991) Where is the wisdom . . .? the poverty of medical evidence, *British Medical Journal* 303: 798–9

Standing M (2005) Perceptions of clinical decision making skills on a developmental journey from student to staff nurse. PhD thesis: University of Kent, Canterbury cited in Standing M (2007) Clinical decision making skills on the developmental journey from student to staff nurse, *Journal of Advanced Nursing* 60(3): 257–69

Standing M (2008) Clinical judgement and decision making in nursing. Nine modes of practice in a revised cognitive continuum, *Journal of Advanced Nursing* 62(1): 124–34

Stone C and Rowles C (2007) Nursing students can help support evidence based practice on clinical nursing units, *Journal of Nursing Management* 15(3): 367–70

Thomas LH, Cullum NA, McColl E, Rousseau N, Soutter J and Steen N (2009) Guidelines in professions allied to medicine (Review). The Cochrane Collaboration. Chichester: John Wiley & Sons. Available at http://www.mrw.interscience.wiley.com/cochrane/clsysrev/articles/CD000349/frame.html (accessed 10 March 2009)

Thompson C (2003) Clinical experience as evidence in evidence-based practice, *Journal of Advanced Nursing* 43(3): 230–7

Thompson C, Cullum N, McCaughan D, Sheldon T and Rayner P (2004) Nurses, information use and clinical decision making – the real world potential for evidence based decisions in nursing, *Evidence-based Nursing* 7: 68–72.

Thompson C, McCaughan D, Cullum N, Sheldon T and Raynor P (2005) Barriers to evidence based practice in primary nursing care, why viewing decision making as context is helpful, *Journal of Advanced Nursing* 52(4): 432–44

Thouless RH and Thouless CR (1953) *Straight and Crooked Thinking* (4th edn). Hoddder and Stoughton: Sevenoaks

Tod A, Palfreyman S and Burke L (2004) Evidence-based practice is a time of opportunity for nursing, *British Journal of Nursing* 13(4): 211–16

Upton D and Upton P (2006a) Knowledge and use of evidence-based practice by allied health and health science professionals in the United Kingdom, *Journal of Allied Health* 35(3): 127–33

Upton D and Upton P (2006b) Development of an evidence based practice questionnaire for nurses, *Journal of Advanced Nursing* 53(4): 454–8

Wakefield AJ, Murch SH, Anthony A and Linnell J (1998) Ileal-lymphoid-nodular hyperplasia, non-specific colitis and pervasive developmental disorder in children, *Lancet* 351: 637–41 (paper now withdrawn)

Zeitz K and McCutcheon H (2003) Evidence based practice – to be or not to be that is the question, *International Journal of Nursing Practice* 9(5): 272–9

Ziebland S, Chapple A, Dumelow C, Evans J, Prinjha S and Rozmovits L (2004) How the internet affects patients' experience of cancer: a qualitative study, *British Medical Journal* 328: 898

Appendix: Useful websites

Individual websites

All accessed on 16 March 2009. All these websites were accurate at the time of going to press. If you are unable to access a link, a simple 'google' search should enable you to access the appropriate website (see below for web base series).

Agree Collaboration is an international collaboration of researchers and policy makers who seek to improve the quality and effectiveness of clinical practice guidelines by establishing a shared framework for their development, reporting and assessment. http://www.agreecollaboration.org/

Bandolier is a useful and easy to read independent journal on evidence based practice. http://www.medicine.ox.ac.uk/bandolier/

Best Treatments is a free evidence-based patient website, based on BMJ's *Clinical Evidence*. It explains chronic conditions and rates the effectiveness of treatments. http://besthealth.bmj.com/btuk/home.jsp

Centre for Evidence Based Medicine (CEBM) is part of a network of centres which review evidence based practice and the factors which impede it. http://www.cebm.net/

Clinical Evidence Clinical Evidence is one of the world's most authoritative medical resources for informing treatment decisions and improving patient care. http://clinicalevidence.bmj.com/ceweb/index.jsp

Clinical Knowledge Summaries is a practical, reliable, evidence-based NHS source. http://cks.library.nhs.uk/home

Cochrane Collaboration for systematic reviews, clinical trials and other sources. http://www.cochrane.org/

Critical Appraisal Skills Programme (CASP) is part of the Public Health Resource Unit, based at the Institute of Health Sciences in Oxford. It produces various appraisal tools for different methodologies. http://www.phru.nhs.uk/Pages/PHD/CASP.htm

Department of Health access to national guidance, benchmarking standards and policy relating to health. http://www.dh.gov.uk/en/index.htm and social care http://www.dh.gov.uk/en/SocialCare/DH_078755

Evidence Based Medicine includes the **What is . . .?** series which explains the terminology and concepts used in EBM. **Gavel** applies EBM principles to key therapeutic areas in primary care. **Clinical Issues in HIV/AIDS** examines the economic, public health, therapeutic and clinical challenges associated with countering HIV/AIDS. http://www.evidence-based-medicine.co.uk/default.html

Health Technology Assessment is part of the National Institute for Health Research (NIHR). It produces independent research information about the effectiveness, costs and broader impact of health care treatments and tests for those who plan, provide or receive care in the NHS. http://www.hta.nhs.uk/

Intute offers a selection of education and research sources by subject area. http://www.intute.ac.uk/ There is a particular site relating to health and social care. http://www.intute.ac.uk/healthandlifesciences/nmaplost.html

Joanna Briggs Institute for Evidence Based Nursing and Midwifery is an international not-for-profit research and development organisation specialising in evidence based resources for health care professionals in nursing, midwifery, medicine and allied health. http://www.joannabriggs.edu.au/about/home.php

Map of Medicine is a clinical information framework designed to make specialised and evidence based practice readily accessible to non-specialists by tracing the patient journey from the first presentation through to final outcome. http://www.mapofmedicine.com/

Monash Institute EBP workbook contains evidence based answers to clinical questions for busy clinicians. http://www.vts.intute.ac.uk/he/tutorial/health

National Institute for Health and Clinical Excellence (NICE) is an independent organisation responsible for providing national guidance on promoting good health and preventing and treating ill health. http://www.nice.org.uk/

National Library for Health (NLH) is a one-stop single search interface for the resources covered by NLH. http://www.library.nhs.uk/evidence/?autoLogin=0

National Guideline Clearinghouse is a public resource for evidence based clinical practice guidelines. http://www.guideline.gov/

Netting the Evidence is intended to facilitate evidence based health care by providing support and access to helpful organisations and useful learning resources, such as an evidence-based virtual library, software and journals. http://www.shef.ac.uk/scharr/ir/netting/

NHS Centre for Reviews and Dissemination, York University, includes Database of Reviews of Effectiveness (DARE), NHS Economic Evaluation Database (NHS EED), and Health Technology Assessment Database. http://www. york.ac.uk/inst/crd/

NMAP is part of the BIOME gateway, providing links to evaluated resources in nursing, midwifery and allied health professions. http://www.intute.ac.uk/ healthandlifesciences/nmaplost.html

Pinakes is a useful subject launch pad (offers an approach for identifying sources relating to specific topic areas. http://www.hw.ac.uk/libwww/irn/ pinakes/pinakes.html

Social Care on line is the UK's most complete range of information and research on all aspects of social care. http://www.scie-socialcareonline.org.uk/ default.asp

Web accessible series

Greenhalgh (1997) How to read a paper. A practical series originally published in the *British Medical Journal* and edited by Trisha Greenhalgh. Also now available as a book from BMJ Publishing Group.

The Medline database, BMJ 1997;315:180–3 (19 July) http://www.bmj.com/ cgi/content/full/315/7101/180

Getting your bearings (deciding what the paper is about), BMJ 1997;315:243–6 (26 July) http://www.bmj.com/cgi/content/full/315/7102/243

Assessing the methodological quality of published papers, BMJ 1997;315 (2 August) http://www.bmj.com/cgi/content/full/315/7103/305

Statistics for the non-statistician. I: Different types of data need different statistical tests, BMJ 1997;315:364–66 (9 August) http://www.bmj.com/cgi/ content/full/315/7104/364

Statistics for the non-statistician. II: 'Significant' relations and their pitfalls,

BMJ 1997;315:422–5 (16 August) http://www.bmj.com/cgi/content/full/315/7105/422

Papers that report drug trials, BMJ 1997;315:480–3 (23 August) http://www.bmj.com/cgi/content/full/315/7106/480

Papers that report diagnostic or screening tests, BMJ 1997;315:540–3 (30 August) http://www.bmj.com/cgi/content/full/315/7107/540

Papers that tell you what things cost (economic analyses), BMJ 1997;315:596–9 (6 September) http://www.bmj.com/cgi/content/full/315/7108/596

Papers that summarise other papers (systematic reviews and meta-analyses), BMJ 1997;315:672–5 (13 September) http://www.bmj.com/cgi/content/full/315/7109/672

Papers that go beyond numbers (qualitative research), BMJ 1997;315:740–3 (20 September) http://www.bmj.com/cgi/content/full/315/7110/740

The Center for Health Evidence: a very good set of **guides to using the literature** were published in the *Journal of the American Medical Association* (*JAMA*) a few years ago and are now available on the Web with clinical scenarios and worked examples of question answering at http://www.cche.net/principles/content_all.asp. Each includes a checklist of questions to use in critical appraisal, and some also include advice about the best Medline search strategy. In detail they cover:

Therapy and prevention http://www.cche.net/principles/content_therapy.asp

Diagnosis http://www.cche.net/principles/content_diagnosis.asp

Harm http://www.cche.net/principles/content_harm.asp

Prognosis http://www.cche.net/principles/content_prognosis.asp

Overview articles http://www.cche.net/principles/content_overview.asp

Clinical decision analyses
http://www.cche.net/principles/content_d_analysis.asp

Clinical practice guidelines
http://www.cche.net/principles/content_p_guideline.asp

Clinical utilisation reviews*
http://www.cche.net/principles/content_u_review.asp

Outcomes of health service research
http://www.cche.net/principles/content_v_outcome.asp

Quality of life measures http://www.cche.net/principles/content_qol.asp

Economic analyses http://www.cche.net/principles/content_e_analysis.asp

Grading health care recommendations
http://www.cche.net/principles/content_grading.asp

Applicability of clinical trials results
http://www.cche.net/principles/content_results.asp

Probability for different diagnoses
http://www.cche.net/principles/content_d_probability.asp

Index